The Journey Through Assessment

In the same series

Food and Your Special Needs Child
Sleep and Your Special Needs Child

The Journey Through Assessment

Help for Parents with a Special Needs Child

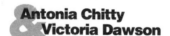

Antonia Chitty & Victoria Dawson

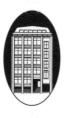

ROBERT HALE • LONDON

ISBN 978-0-7198-0789-3

Robert Hale Limited
Clerkenwell House
Clerkenwell Green
London EC1R 0HT

www.halebooks.com

2 4 6 8 10 9 7 5 3 1

Typeset by Eurodesign
Printed in the UK by the Berforts Group

Contents

Acknowledgements

This book could not have been written without the help and support of a number of people. We would like to offer our sincere thanks to the many parents who took the time to share their experiences of assessment with us. Their insight has allowed us to provide real-life case studies and to share strategies that will hopefully help to support other families in similar situations.

We would also like to thank the numerous professionals who offered their support and advice throughout the book:

Dr Kairen Cullen, an educational psychologist who has worked with many children and their families to offer guidance around learning. Dr Cullen is frequently featured in the national media as an expert in her field and we thank her for offering her time to our research. More details about Dr Cullen may be found on the British Psychological Society website at www.bps.org.uk and the Association of Child Psychologists in Private Practice website at www.achippp.org.uk.

Sue Atkins, a parenting expert whose vision is to empower and inspire parents, gave up her valuable time to provide input for our book. Sue is a former deputy head, writer, speaker and parenting coach, and perhaps most importantly is also a parent herself. To learn more about her work log on to www.sueatkinsparentingcoach.com.

Dr Louise Langman is a chartered clinical psychologist and has an expertise in family therapy. Dr Langman also specializes in autism spectrum disorders and offers support directly to parents as well as undertaking medico-legal work. More details about Dr Langman can be found at www.achippp.org.uk/directory/psychologist/228.

Vicky Robinson is a children's occupational therapist who specializes in motor co-ordination and sensory processing issues. Her website can be found at www.enabletherapy.co.uk. Vicky works in partnership with children, parents and families to support them in achieving their goals.

Chapter 1
Introduction

Are you concerned about your child? Right now, you may be feeling scared, anxious or uncertain. If you believe that there is something wrong with your child, but have yet to get a diagnosis, this book is for you. It can feel isolating if your child is being assessed for special needs: you can feel bewildered by the education and health systems. You may also have difficult feelings to deal with from denial to blame, guilt to desperation. It can put a strain on your relationships with your partner or other family members. You can feel like you are struggling to look after your other children. Other parents go through all this too: read this book and you won't feel so alone.

With one in every ten children now being diagnosed with dyslexia and one in a hundred with autism, the journey of assessment and diagnosis is becoming a familiar path for many families. Having a child assessed for an additional need can put a strain on your family. This book looks at the issues that you might face along the way and how to overcome these.

Most importantly we also aim to focus on the positives that assessment and diagnosis can bring for you and your child. Use the book as a tool to help you talk about your child, the assessment process and how you are feeling.

This book is written for parents who suspect their child has 'special needs', special educational needs, additional needs or a disability, but just what is meant by those terms?

A disability is something that limits someone. It can be:

✓ physical
✓ cognitive
✓ mental
✓ sensory
✓ emotional
✓ developmental

Often disability is due to an impairment in the sense of a problem in body function or structure This may cause someone to have difficulty in doing things, or restrict that person from taking part in activities. According to the World Health Organization, '... disability is a complex phenomenon, reflecting an interaction between features of a person's body and features of the society in which he or she lives.'

According to the Department for Education, pupils with special educational needs have learning difficulties or disabilities that make it harder for them to learn than most pupils of their age.

The most common types of special educational needs are autism spectrum disorder and moderate learning difficulties.

Special educational needs can be classified as:

✓ a specific learning disability
✓ a moderate learning disability
✓ a severe learning disability
✓ profound and multiple learning disabilities
✓ behavioural, emotional and social difficulties
✓ speech, language and communication needs
✓ a hearing impairment
✓ a visual impairment
✓ a multi-sensory impairment
✓ a physical disability
✓ autism spectrum disorder

One in five school-age children in England have special educational needs. Boys are more likely to have a statement of special educational needs than girls.

Parent coach Sue Atkins gives her own perspective on what 'special needs' means:

❝ *'Special Needs' is like an umbrella sheltering and hiding a huge collection of diagnoses underneath. Children with 'special' or 'different' needs may have trouble paying attention, have profound learning difficulties or be gifted, or they may have a food allergy, be terminally ill or have a stammer. The vastness of the term can be confusing and bewildering.*

*Special need is commonly defined by what your child
can't do – by milestones unmet, foods banned, activities
avoided and experiences denied. These minuses can hit you
as a family really hard and may make 'special needs' seem
like a tragic designation or a millstone around everyone's
neck. But I believe that a label should not limit a child's
potential and I see every child as a way to find a new opportunity to explore their potential in a new or different way that
hasn't yet been tried.* **"**

Whatever condition your child has, assessment can be the first step in
getting the help they need. Some conditions can be spotted at birth,
such as Down's syndrome or cerebral palsy, but even if you or the
doctor can clearly see that there is an issue, you are still likely to have
to wait for tests to be carried out in the days and weeks after your
child's birth for a definite diagnosis. This wait can be hard to deal
with as you come to terms with a different future for your child to the
one you imagined while they were in the womb.

Other conditions become evident as your child grows, perhaps if
their development is slower than expected. Sensory impairments,
developmental delay and conditions on the autism spectrum often
show up in this way. You can feel frustrated that you have concerns
about your child's development, you might be unsure where to turn,
or you may be worried that professionals are not taking your concerns
seriously. Alternatively, it may be that the first suggestion that your
child has a problem comes out of the blue at a routine health check or
from a child care professional. Either way, it can take some time to get
a diagnosis, and the process can be stressful for you as a parent.

Nonetheless, assessment and diagnosis are the first step towards
helping your child. They can be key to accessing appropriate medical
care, aids, physical and occupational therapy, or learning support at
school. When it seems like assessment is taking forever, remember
that this means your child is getting a thorough investigation. It may
be that a number of different professionals and specialist equipment
are required to give results which are likely to be reviewed and
brought together into a diagnosis by a paediatric consultant. The
consultant should then take time to explain to you about what the test

results mean, the implications for your child, their care and their future.

When it is suspected that your child may have an additional need it can feel like your world has fallen apart. This book will help you access the support you need as a parent as you support your child. You will learn about avoidable problems and get help to guide you through the troublesome times that can't be avoided.

In Chapter 2, you can start by finding out more about sharing concerns. If you have concerns about your child, this chapter will help you identify as specifically as possible your concerns and what they are based on. Noting down evidence of your concerns can help you get the outcome you want from your first meeting with a health care professional. In this chapter you can also explore issues around sharing your concerns with your partner and what to do if your partner doesn't share your concerns. You will get information on who to speak to about your concerns and the professionals that can help. Plus, read tips on how to make sure that you share your concerns with professionals effectively.

If you are in a situation where someone else has raised concerns about your child that you don't share, try reading Chapter 3. Whether your partner, a professional, a friend or stranger has suggested that you might want to seek help for your child, read this chapter for advice about what to do next. You will discover the importance of acknowledging the concern and learn how to monitor the issue. You can read about other parents in this situation, including those who have decided against a diagnosis or intervention.

In Chapter 4 you can learn all about assessment and what it will involve. Discover tips on preparing your child for assessment, and also on preparing yourself both in a practical way and emotionally. You can read case studies about parents and their experiences of different assessments and get information from professionals, from paediatricians to educational psychologists, on different assessments. Vitally, you can learn how to celebrate your child's functioning in the assessment, making it a positive experience.

Next, get tips and advice on working in partnership with professionals. Chapter 5 explains how professionals should support families through assessment and you can read case studies of positive experiences of working in partnership. You'll learn practical tips that have been used by other parents to make any appointment easier, and learn how to be clear about developing a good working relationship. Discover which professionals you might meet to help with your child's educational needs. Plus, if things don't go well, you can get advice on how to complain.

Depending on your views, you may be keen to hear the name of your child's condition, or you may be devastated by news worse than you had hoped for. In Chapter 6 you will get advice on how to cope when receiving difficult news. Learn about the range of feelings that you may go through. Explore how you and your partner or other family members may react differently, and how to deal with that. You can also get advice on what to do if you need to share difficult news resulting from the diagnosis with your child. Plus, there is also advice on sharing news of the diagnosis with your child's school or other services.

Chapter 7 is packed with practical tips to help you following a diagnosis. As you learn about your child's condition, this chapter helps with ways to stay organized and remember appointments and important information. Find out about the stages you might go through in coming to terms with your child's diagnosis, and get tips on gathering helpful information. Explore the options available if you need someone to talk to for emotional support, and discover support groups that might help on- and offline.

In Chapter 8, you can start moving on from your child's diagnosis with positive strategies to minimize their difficulties: set small achievable targets and celebrate your child's successes. You will discover who can help you with this and how to create opportunities to maximize your child's strengths.

Moving on from diagnosis, Chapter 9 helps you deal with some of the less positive aspects of having a child with special needs. Get tips on how to deal with stress, and how to communicate your feelings about diagnosis rather than bottling them up. Read advice on how to support other family members to move on. Find out how to cope if your child is not making progress, and read how other parents enjoy their children. This chapter also outlines how to ensure that your child is supported in school and what to do if you have concerns.

Chapter 10 looks at the positives about assessment and diagnosis. Reflect back on the positives that the assessment has brought to your child and your family. Consider the help your child now has, the positive people you have met and the qualities you have developed as a result of this experience. Read about how other parents' lives have changed in unexpected ways as a result of a diagnosis of special educational needs or disability, and hear from parents writing about their journey.

Chapter 2
Sharing Concerns

Nobody knows a child better than his/her parent. You really are the expert on your own son or daughter. If you have a concern about your child it is important that you act upon it. Sharing concerns around your child can be a very daunting task. Reading the experiences of other parents may help you to realize that you are not alone and give you the confidence to move the assessment process forward if necessary.

This chapter will explore:

✓ identifying what your concerns are
✓ finding evidence to support your concerns
✓ considering areas that may cause concerns
✓ sharing concerns with others effectively

Concerned about being concerned?

Being a parent can be extremely stressful and is a huge responsibility. As a caring mother or father you want your child to reach their full potential, whatever that may be. You know your child better than anybody else in the world and are best placed to pick up any concerns around your child at an early stage. If you have a concern about your child and professionals don't appear to share this concern you can begin to question your own judgment. Sometimes as parents we have a gut feeling that something isn't quite right with our child's development yet we feel that we may be causing a fuss or even being neurotic.

Julie was worried about her daughter's vision yet felt that she was being labelled an overprotective first-time mother. She tells us:

" *Jess was a difficult baby right from the start. I frequently went to the health visitor for advice only to be told that she was fine* *and that this is how babies are. I started to feel like I was becoming a nuisance to be honest and decided to keep my worries to myself. When she got to twelve months, however, I noticed that her eyes would turn upwards when she tried to focus on things. This was something that I simply couldn't ignore. I took her to the GP who referred us to a local children's hospital. Jess went through the most ridiculous assessment process I have ever encountered. They asked her to match letters, at twelve months old she had no concept of matching whatsoever! They also asked her to look at and iden-tify pictures at a distance, again she couldn't achieve this task. Jess was discharged from the hospital and was described as being 'uncooperative'. I didn't feel strong enough at this time to challenge the way the assessment was conducted so I just accepted that everything was fine, even though I knew that it wasn't. Six months later I was walking past an opticians and I decided to take Jess in and ask for her to be examined. The optician was lovely and saw her straight away. The optician's face as she examined Jess said it all, she informed me that Jess had a significant visual impairment and needed to be seen by specialists as soon as possible. A referral was made to another hospital and she got the treatment that she needed. My concerns were right, I wasn't a neurotic mother and I didn't have a difficult child! My advice to other parents who have concerns is to have confidence in yourself. If you think there is something amiss then keep at the professionals.* **"**

Julie's story highlights how parental concern is often right. If you are worried about your child it is important that you seek help and advice for your child's sake.

What are your concerns?

Sometimes it is difficult to pinpoint exactly what you are concerned about; in other cases it is obvious. For example, Joanne knew that her son's speech was delayed and that a referral to the speech therapy service would be appropriate.

❝ *Reece is the youngest of three children. I'm an early years teacher so know all about developmental stages. I was very aware that Reece's expressive language was delayed, he had only around ten words at the age of two. He was, however, very good at getting his needs met and relied heavily on gesturing and vocalization. I did initially put it down to being the youngest and the fact that we had all babied him but he failed to make significant progress over the next few months and so I requested a referral to the Speech and Language Therapist via my health visitor. We attended some classes held in a local children's centre and I'm delighted to say that Reece has made excellent progress and that his language is now age appropriate.* **❞**

Rachel, in contrast, had concerns about her son in a number of developmental areas including his communication skills, play skills and behaviour.

❝ *I initially raised concerns about Harry's development with my health visitor when he was ten months old. She basically told me that I was being a paranoid mother! I was told that he was a second child, and a boy, so he was going to develop at a slower rate than my daughter. I felt that my concerns weren't listened to. Harry was making no attempt to crawl and he was demonstrating self-stimulatory behaviours such as rocking and head-banging, he also showed little interest in toys. We raised concerns again at thirteen months, which were taken seriously this time and the assessment process began. Harry got a formal diagnosis of Autism and Global Developmental Delay at the age of twenty-six months.* **❞**

Though Rachel unfortunately found that her initial concerns were not acknowledged, her persistence resulted in an assessment being carried out and her son receiving the appropriate diagnosis and support. It is important that if you feel that you have not been listened to you do seek further advice and request a second opinion if necessary.

Dr Kairen Cullen is an educational psychologist and author of the book *Introducing Child Psychology*. Dr Cullen has worked with many families who have concerns around their child's functioning. She tells us:

ff *Communication is the key to sharing concerns. Generally speaking the first port of call will be the class teacher. There is a whole system in school for sharing concerns, which can include the SENCO (Special Educational Needs Co-ordinator) and head teacher. If a parent feels that their concerns are not being heard, putting them in writing can be helpful. Many local authorities have parent support workers who may act as advocates for parents. The home/school link should be a partnership in order for children to have a successful educational experience. The school of course has a part to play in this and should raise concerns with parents as soon as possible if they believe a child may need assessing.* **ff**

Areas for concern

There are a number of areas that can cause concern for parents with regard to their children. Below is a list of areas that you may wish to consider when attempting to pinpoint your concerns. Identifying what your specific concerns are at this stage is very helpful as it will allow you to draw together all the information that you require in order to share your concerns effectively with a professional. It will also help to ensure that your child is referred to the appropriate agent for assessment if necessary.

Speech and language skills

You may be concerned that your child's language is not developing as quickly as it should. There may be specific problems with your child's speech in terms of stammering or perhaps they are struggling to make specific sounds. If you have concerns around your child's understanding this should also be mentioned.

Speech and language therapists also assess as part of the diagnostic team for social communication disorders such as autism and Asperger's syndrome.

Gross motor skills

Gross motor skills refer to any of the skills used in moving the large muscles in the body: the legs, arms and torso. Walking, climbing, jumping and crawling are all examples of gross motor skills. A child who is presenting with gross motor skills difficulties may not be able to do these tasks at an age appropriate level or when performing these tasks they may become unsteady, appearing to be clumsy. Physiotherapists assess children for concerns around gross motor skills.

Fine motor skills

Fine motor skills refer to the small movements made to perform tasks such as holding a pencil or threading beads. Some children have difficulties in this area and will need an assessment by an occupational therapist (OT).

Cognitive difficulties

Some children have delayed thinking, learning and problem-solving skills. If you are concerned about your child's cognitive skills your nursery/school Special Educational Needs Co-ordinator (SENCO) will be able to offer you advice about who to refer to if necessary.

Emotional difficulties

Emotional problems can include children having anxiety issues, irrational fears and behavioural difficulties. A referral to your local CAMHS service may be appropriate. CAMHS means Child and Adolescent Mental Health Services and is an NHS service.

Behavioural Issues

At some point all children demonstrate some challenging behaviour. If, however, the behaviour is becoming progressively worse no matter what you try and you are finding it difficult to identify triggers for the behaviour, an assessment may be necessary. Behaviour issues can include withdrawn behaviour as well as aggressive behaviour. Your local authority may have a specialist behaviour support service, or a referral to CAMHS may be appropriate.

Sensory impairment

Some children have sensory impairment such as hearing impairments and visual impairments. If you are concerned about your child's vision or hearing it is important that you get it checked out. Other forms of sensory impairment include problems with sense of taste, smell, touch and spatial awareness. There are sensory impairment teams based within local authorities who have specialist teachers and occupational therapists trained to work with children with sensory issues.

Specific learning difficulties

Some children have specific learning difficulties such as dyslexia. If you are concerned about your child's education initially speak with the school. Ask yourself what area of their learning you are worried about. Is it that they are struggling in particular curriculum areas such as reading, writing or spelling? Or are you concerned about their general abilities? 'Specific learning difficulties' describes a group of conditions including dyspraxia, dyscalculia and dysgraphia. Dyspraxia is a co-ordination disorder, dyscalculia occurs when a child finds learning around numbers challenging and dysgraphia may be diagnosed when a child has difficulty putting their thoughts down on paper.

Multiple concerns

It may be that you are concerned about your child in a number of different areas, for example their speech, behaviour and fine motor skills. It is important that you identify all the areas that you are concerned about so that the appropriate referral can be made.

Health issues

Are you worried about any aspects of your child's health? Areas that may cause concern are feeding and swallowing issues, breathing difficulties, regular illnesses, weight gain or loss or sleep issues.

Having read this list, in the space below write down the areas of concern that you have around your child:

1. ....
....
....

2. ....
....
....

3. ....
....
....

4. ....
....
....

5. ....
....
....

Describing concerns

Having identified your concerns it is now time to analyze them so that you can decide whether you do need to be pursuing an assessment for your child and so that you can present the information clearly to professionals.

When you take your concerns to a practitioner it is important that you describe very clearly what you are concerned about. It is helpful, therefore, if before your appointment you carefully consider the information that you are going to share with them to highlight your concerns.

John, whose son Jake has developmental delay says, 'Whenever I went to see a professional about my children I always ended up coming away feeling that I'd only told them half a story. I now make sure I write everything down that I want to get across at the appointment.'

Sonya is a specialist teacher and tells us:

" *Parents often attend appointments with me and just tell me that there is 'something wrong' with their child. It can then take me a long time to get to the bottom of their concerns and to identify the appropriate pathway for them. It is really helpful when parents can give me an indication of the areas that they are concerned about and evidence this with some examples. So one parent was worried about her son's frequent falling down and apparent clumsiness; she recorded him on her mobile phone and she could then show me during the appointment exactly what she meant. It was immediately apparent to me that this child needed a referral on to a physiotherapist and I could action this straight away.* "

Now that you have identified the general areas of concern it is important that you be as specific as possible about what exactly you are concerned about. Taking time now to consider in depth each area that is concerning you will mean that you find it much easier to share this with others.

Start by thinking about the one issue that causes you the most concern. And use the grid below to help you to analyze exactly what your worry is. Providing an example of the concern is also very useful and it will help you to illustrate to the listener exactly what you mean.

A number of examples have been completed for you so that you can see the kind of information that it will be useful to share: see page 24.

Difficulties identifying concerns

If you have concerns around your child but are finding it difficult to specifically identify what they are, it may be useful to speak to others. If you have a partner or family member who is supportive then try to set aside some time to specifically discuss your concerns. It is important that this time is free from interruptions so that you can really focus on your conversations.

Try to think of examples of the issues that cause concern and write them down. Identifying examples may help you to decipher exactly what it is about these incidents that make them concerning.

If your child attends nursery or school it would be worth speaking to staff at the setting to find out whether they have any concerns. Sometimes children present differently in different environments. You should share with the staff what your concerns are, giving them examples and see if they have noticed anything similar happening while your child is with them. If the staff in the setting don't share your concerns then make a note of this as it is useful information to pass on when sharing your concerns with another professional.

Jody tells us:

" *I knew very early on that there was a problem with my child. However, I think deep down you still pray that you will be told that there is nothing 'wrong' and it is something like a parenting problem, as this is easier to fix. The biggest piece of advice I can give to any parent at this stage is to talk. If you can't go to supportive family members or friends, access local support groups or national organizations. I found the SEN chat forum on Netmums really valuable; it enabled me to talk about my concerns to other parents who were in a similar position.* "

Worried about your child?

All children, at some point in their lives, cause their parents concern. The question is whether the concerns you have warrant assessment from professionals. Children change and develop all the time and it may be that the concern you have about your child right now will have rectified itself in six months' time without the need for intervention.

The difficulty for any parent is deciding how long to wait before seeking an assessment. It is always useful to speak to a practitioner and share your concerns. They are best placed to advise whether assessment would be the appropriate form of action. Some children are assessed and the assessment outcome suggests that no intervention is required as, over the period of assessment, the child has made sufficient progress. Parents often worry that their child will be incorrectly

Area of concern	Specific concern	First noticed concern	Example
Behaviour	John will bang his head repeatedly on hard surfaces and doesn't seem to feel any pain	At the age of two years	When I turned the TV off last night he repeatedly banged his head on the floor, no comfort helped, even putting the TV back on didn't help
Speech and language	Abigail's speech is very unclear. You can hear some key words but otherwise it is hard to understand her	Always been unclear since she started speaking at about eighteen months	She was asking me for a drink of water and a biscuit. The only word I could make out was 'water', which wasn't clear, she then led me by the hand to show me
Learning	Leon is finding reading very challenging and his writing is unclear	He enjoyed sharing books until he was five years old and started full-time school. He now gets very upset and seems aware of his difficulties	He got frustrated when reading books last night and threw them. He is not forming the letters of the alphabet still and reverses letters such as p, b and d
Emotional difficulties	Tilly is very anxious. She does a lot of compulsive checking. She also frequently gets out of bed to check where family members are. Her sleep is very poor	Always been anxious but has started to get worse since she moved to secondary school	Tilly has to check before we leave the house that all electrical items are switched off. She has a routine of touching certain objects in the house before she leaves such as her teddy, the radiator cover in the hallway and a picture on the wall

Area of concern	Specific concern	First noticed concern	Example

diagnosed or labelled once the assessment process begins. If this is causing you concern share this with a practitioner.

If you are concerned enough about your child to be reading this book it is highly likely that it is time to share these concerns. There is a huge push in the UK for early intervention for children with additional needs. Research has shown that early intervention allows children and their families to use the available support more efficiently, with greater long-term benefits for all involved.

Relationships and Communication

It can be hugely stressful if you suspect that your child has a special need. It is important that those around you are supportive, though at times it can be those closest to you that cause you the greatest amount of stress.

Parents' experiences of sharing concerns can be very mixed, depending on your circumstances. Some parents may live apart and this can cause an added pressure on a relationship that may already be fragile. Simon tells us, 'I'm really concerned about my daughter. Isabelle is four years old and I suspect she is on the autism spectrum. She lives with her mum as we have recently divorced. I have tried to speak to her mother about this but she will not acknowledge any difficulties.'

Other parents shared experiences of being together as a couple but feeling very differently about their child's needs. Sally says:

" *I know that Thomas has problems. He is struggling to mix with other children and his language is delayed. His teacher at school is beginning to have concerns yet my partner will not accept that there are any difficulties at all. I'm not sure whether he is in denial or it is because he works away a lot and he doesn't see the full extent of what is happening. His attitude is that he was just the same as Thomas as a child and his mother backs him up with this. I'm at a loss as to know what to do now!* **"**

Having different feelings from your child's other parent is not unusual but it does make the whole experience of initiating assessment much more difficult. We are all individuals and deal with emotional issues in our own way. There may be many reasons why the other parent doesn't share a concern about a child, including denial.

Emotions can run very high when talking about a child's difficulties. Both parents usually want what is best for their child; the difficulty is trying to negotiate in order to find an outcome that is acceptable to both parents *and* has the child's best interests at the fore.

Relationships with other family members can also be put under pressure. Many families shared with us the impact of well-meaning grandparents who made attempts to offer support but sometimes got it very wrong! Julie says:

" *My mother thinks she is being helpful but really she isn't. Leo has a hearing impairment, which was picked up fairly early on. My mum has been in denial ever since. She doesn't realize that sometimes I find her 'help' incredibly offensive and draining. She still has no concerns around Leo's hearing and refuses to learn to sign as she is convinced it is unnecessary as he can hear perfectly well.* **"**

If you have concerns around your child's development it is important that you action these as appropriate. When others don't share your concerns it can be very difficult and you begin to question your own judgment. If in doubt seek advice from a health or education professional.

Share the information that you put together in the table on page 25 with those who do not share your worries. This may help them to see more clearly what you are concerned about. It may also help to open up some important dialogue around concerns and your child's functioning. Remember that you all love and care for your child.

Some families find that if they can't agree about concerns then counselling is an option that needs to be explored. If you feel that your relationship does need some support you can ask your GP to refer you to a counsellor. Some organizations provide free counselling to their staff so if you are employed it is worth checking to see whether this is available. Or alternatively you can pay to see a counsellor privately. Talking to somebody who isn't emotionally involved can be difficult at first but also very beneficial.

Lynn Wilshaw is a Relate counsellor and she advises:

" *If you and your partner have different views about your child and their needs this can very easily lead to conflict. If you are having issues within your relationship counselling can help you to explore each other's feelings and perspectives. Counselling isn't about offering you advice but about exploring the emotional effects of sharing your concerns about your child with each other. It can help you to address how you communicate with each other and enable you to develop and enhance these skills.* **"**

Lynn offers advice about what to look for when choosing a counsellor: 'You must feel comfortable with the counsellor that you choose. You should make telephone contact with a number of counsellors initially if you are going to go privately and ask them questions about their experience and qualifications. Which counsellor makes you feel at ease and relaxed?'

Read more about counselling and the emotional issues raised by the assessment process in Chapters 6, 7 and 9.

Sharing concerns with professionals

Having identified your concerns and shared them with appropriate family members, the next step is to share them with the professionals. This can sometimes seem a big step to take and it may also make your concern appear to be more 'real'.

There are a huge range of professionals involved with children's assessments and it is little wonder that parents often feel overwhelmed regarding whom to approach with their concerns. If your child is under five years old you should contact your health visitor initially. If they attend nursery or pre-school you should also speak to professionals there regarding your worries. Early years settings have SENCOs who can offer you support and advice as appropriate.

If your child is over five years old you should contact your GP, a school nurse or a SENCO within your child's school and they should be able to help you to identify the appropriate referral route.

It is important that the professional makes time to hear your concerns. Request an appointment so that you can sit down with the practitioner and share information effectively. This will ensure you get their full attention and that you aren't interrupted.

Preparing to share information

You may initially feel nervous about meeting with a professional; always remember that you are the expert on your child. Professionals are there to help and support you and your child. The professional may be an expert in their field but you also bring vital parenting expertise to the meeting. Julie reminds us, 'Don't be afraid of the professionals. They probably know more about your child's condition than you do, but they don't know more about your child, or your child's individual needs.'

It may help you to feel more confident if you take some time to prepare for the meeting.

Consider the following:

✓ What do you want the professional to understand about your child/family?
✓ What are the key concerns you have to share?
✓ What do you want the outcome of the meeting to be?

Considering these questions will give you a clearer idea of what you are hoping to achieve from the meeting and help you to be more focused.

Where to meet

Some professionals may be able to offer you a home visit to discuss your concerns. Consider whether you would find it easier to meet in your home environment than a more clinical setting.

Advantages of meeting at home include:

✓ You don't have to factor in travel time

✓ There are no transport or parking issues
✓ You may feel more at ease in your own surroundings

Disadvantages of meeting at home can include:

✓ You may become distracted by visitors or the phone ringing
✓ You may feel stressed about whether your home is tidy enough
✓ Some parents do not want neighbours to see 'officials' going to the house for fear of gossip

Annette says, 'In the early days I would rush around trying to be Superwoman, making sure the house, my child and myself were spotless. I have learned over the years to be more relaxed about assessments and now have the attitude that they take me as they find me!' If you are not offered a home visit and would prefer one then do ask whether this is an option. If you are offered a home visit yet would prefer to meet in a different setting it is important that you request this. You must feel as comfortable as possible in the meeting's surroundings.

Who should attend?

If possible, it is always helpful to attend meetings with somebody else to support you. This can make you feel more confident and they can remind you of anything that you may have forgotten to mention. It is quite common after a meeting to forget parts of what was said, and a supportive friend or family member will act as another set of ears for you and may well remember those details that have slipped your mind.

Michelle advises, 'It really helps if you can take someone else with you, be it a friend, a family member or someone from the parent partnership organization. Their perspective on what is discussed can often be different to your own.'

If you do take somebody with you ensure that it is somebody who will be supportive. You don't want to have to worry that they are going to lose their temper or contradict what you are saying.

If you can't find anybody to attend the meeting with you, you may wish to consider using a recording device within the meeting (with the professional's consent, of course). Explain to them that you are concerned that you may forget what is said afterwards. On another note, a recording of the session is a great way of informing other people of what has happened during the meeting rather than you having to regularly repeat the information, which is something that some parents can find hugely emotionally draining. Many smart-phones now have a voice recorder.

Collecting thoughts

It can be a useful but difficult exercise to write down your child's history to date. Often parents are asked to share this information at each appointment that they have with a new practitioner. This can be extremely emotionally draining, particularly if your child has had a traumatic history. Many parents find it useful to write all of this infor-mation down so that they don't have to relive those painful memories and can simply hand over the information to be read. Or if you do feel able to verbally share the information with the professional it may act as a visual aid so that you don't forget any important details.

The table below can act as a template for you to record any infor-mation that practitioners may need to know: see page 32.

Organizing paperwork

Unfortunately assessment generally creates a huge amount of paper-work and it is easy to get quickly overwhelmed by this. Chloe tells us, 'I keep a file for my child's paperwork and regularly go through it and remove old documentation and replace it with up to date letters and reports.'

Getting into good habits early on makes it much easier as the assessment evolves. Rachel says:

“ *Keeping records or diaries is really important. Have a specific diary that you use for your child to write things into as you will need to look back at it to find out information such as dates of appointments. You can also use the diary to monitor your child's progress and to see if there are any patterns in their behaviour.* **”**

Child's name:	
DOB:	
Any difficulties in pregnancy:	
Any difficulties at birth:	
Any medication/allergies:	
General health and well-being:	
Details of any other professionals involved:	
School/nursery:	
Current concerns around your child:	
Strengths of your child:	

While it can seem an onerous task keeping your paperwork in order, Simone explains the positive side of it:

❝ *We kept a folder with dividers for each professional involved with Charlie. We kept copies of reports that they had produced and also our notes from meetings that we attended. My advice to other parents is to keep everything and keep as much of it in writing as possible. It's often nice to look back. When you first get reports and see your child's difficulties being described in black and white, it is really, really difficult. However, seven years later it's amazing to look back and see the progress he has made.* **❞**

The meeting

Being fully prepared for a meeting helps you to feel more in control. Here are some tips to make this an easier experience:

- ✓ If the meeting is outside your home always make sure you know where you are going
- ✓ Ask for the professional's telephone number, just in case you need to contact them regarding the arrangements for any reason
- ✓ Dress in a way that makes you feel comfortable; nobody is judging you on your appearance
- ✓ Take notes with you and use them throughout the session. They are there for you to refer to
- ✓ Take some tissues. You may think that you are going to be fine during the meeting but sometimes it can be very emotional speaking about your child's needs
- ✓ If you do feel upset during the meeting explain this to the practitioner
- ✓ Take some deep breaths to help you to keep calm
- ✓ If the outcome of the meeting is not what you hoped for, don't be afraid to ask for a second opinion
- ✓ Write down a list of all the questions that you would like to be answered prior to the meeting and make sure in the meeting that everything has been covered

✓ Ask questions; if there is something that you aren't sure about then you must ask

✓ Before you leave make sure that you find out what will happen next. So, for example, will you need to attend a further meeting? Or will you get an appointment letter to go to the hospital? Also ask for an indication of how long you can expect to wait until you hear something about the next stage of the process – this will stop you worrying if you don't hear immediately

Advice from practitioners

Sonya works as a specialist teacher and meets with parents on a daily basis who have concerns around their child's development. She tells us,

I think that the initial meeting prior to initiating assessment is very important for both parent and practitioner. This is an opportunity to develop a good working relationship and to do the very best for that child. Although it possibly sounds ridiculous, professionals get nervous too at these meetings. Even though I have done this job for the last fifteen years, it gets no easier trying to find the right words to use when a parent begins the journey of assessment with their child. As far as advice to parents is concerned I would say to go with your gut instinct; if you think that something is amiss then it needs to be explored. Pinpoint exactly what it is that you would like professionals to be aware of. Don't be afraid of us, we are here to help you. I appreciate that it is an emotionally difficult time for parents and I really do want to make things as easy as possible; good communication is the key and that is a two-way process. If I get something wrong then please tell me and give me the opportunity to put it right.

In summary

Parenting is a very difficult job, and when you feel that your child is not developing typically the stress can be tremendous. Analyzing exactly what it is that you are concerned about will help you to develop a clearer thought pattern around the problem. Identifying people in your life who can support you through the assessment process if necessary is extremely helpful. Good communication is key to sharing information about worries and concerns. Write down any questions that you may have and use written notes to prompt you in meetings. Remind yourself that you are doing a fantastic job as a parent and that you are the expert on your child.

Chapter 3
Acknowledging Concerns

As we discussed in the last chapter, nobody knows a child better than a parent or primary caregiver. When somebody else raises a concern about your child's development or functioning it can therefore be very upsetting, particularly if you don't share their concern.

This chapter will explore:

✓ Who may highlight concerns and for what reason
✓ How you may feel about these concerns being raised about your child
✓ How to deal with these difficult conversations
✓ Monitoring concerns if appropriate

We will also include case studies from parents who have not had concerns about their child's development and have experienced others expressing concern and examine how they have handled this situation.

Gina's son is seven years old and his teacher recently expressed concerns around his physical skills. She tells us:

" I've always encouraged friends to go along the diagnosis route, always given the advice that a label doesn't change who your child is, that they are still the same great kid, label or no label. I firmly believe that there is no shame in getting a condition named and that it is good to know what you are dealing with so that you can get your child the best possible help. I still hold by that but I guess being in the situation myself has made it clearer that there are shades of grey, it's not all black and white at all. I guess my only advice would be to put your child's well-being right at the centre of any decision you make – but I am sure any parent would do that anyway. "

Who may express a concern?

As we explored in the previous chapter parents can have many different concerns about their child's development. These can range from physical to communication difficulties or from behaviour to emotional issues. Throughout childhood a variety of professionals will assess your child both formally and informally.

Midwives

Assessment begins in the womb with mothers being invited to attend regular appointments and being offered scans of their baby. Scans give the opportunity to assess growth and the well-being of the baby. Measurements can be taken and the amount of amniotic fluid around baby can be assessed.

Children are also assessed for well-being immediately after birth when a physical examination is carried out. Newborn babies are generally assessed using the APGAR score, which is a basic physiological assessment of the vital functions. The midwives will also be informally observing newborns; hearing tests are offered and a midwife should also offer support after the birth, when informal assessment of the baby and mother is continued. It's amazing to think that all this assessment takes place so soon after birth!

If you are worried about the assessments that are taking place ask practitioners to explain to you what they are assessing. Sometimes not knowing exactly why assessments are taking place can make you feel agitated when in actual fact it may be something very routine that is happening.

Health visitors

Once the midwife has discharged the family, usually around ten days after the birth, the health visitor generally takes over. The health visitor's role in the early years is an extremely important one. A health visitor is a registered nurse or midwife who has undertaken further training and his/her aim is to improve the health and well-being of families and their children. They support a family until a child's fifth birthday. They can be a useful resource for information and can advise on a range of important issues such as health, feeding and sleeping difficulties.

Health visitors also assess children and if you have concerns around any aspect of your pre-school child's development these should be shared. The health visitor asks questions about the child's functioning and makes observations as well as measuring height, weight and head circumference. Health visitors may identify a concern around a child's functioning during these assessments. If they do share a concern with you it can be shocking if you have not been aware of anything being amiss yourself.

Julie says:

" *I took my son to his nine-month assessment recently to see the health visitor. I was very happy with his development, he's a lovely little boy and is reaching all his developmental milestones. When I arrived it wasn't how I expected it would be for a start and this made me feel uneasy. When I had my older daughter the assessments were carried out at home; this one was carried out at the local children's centre. I suppose I was already feeling a bit anxious as I was out of my comfort zone. On arrival there were three members of staff and I didn't know any of them. I asked where my health visitor was and they said she wasn't covering clinic that day. I was taken into a large room where there were other parents and babies. It soon became clear that the assessment was going to take place in here, which didn't feel very comfortable to me. I undressed Sam as they wanted to take his measurements and I became aware that after measuring his head two of the professionals were discussing him in hushed voices. I knew that they thought something was wrong and started to feel quite tearful. I was approached in front of the other parents and told that his head measurements were very large and they wanted to measure him again to check that they were accurate. I explained that I'd already seen my GP about his head as it was still a little misshapen following birth and she'd assured me that it was fine. I felt like they didn't listen to what I was saying at all and just carried on measuring him and saying that the measurements were concerning. They told me that I must see my GP straight away and give her the details of the measurements so that she could refer us on if necessary. I felt really angry about the way this news was shared with me, in front of other mothers in the neighbourhood. I don't want to discuss my child in front of anyone else and I did actually complete an evaluation form of the session and explained that parents should be able to have an assessment in a confidential situation. After all, you wouldn't expect a doctor to discuss your symptoms in a waiting room would you? I did get Sam checked out again and there was nothing wrong with his head. Although I didn't share their concerns I have to admit it did get me doubting myself and my GP.* 〃

Health visitors are highly experienced practitioners who are well placed to pick up issues early on. Research shows that early intervention is most successful as the earlier that issues are picked up the more easily they can be addressed. If your health visitor does pick up on an issue that you haven't been concerned about ask for an appointment to discuss it in detail. Julie's experience was compounded by the fact that the feedback was given in a public space – you should always be offered a confidential space to discuss your child. If this is not offered then you should explain to the professional that the content of the discussion is personal and that you would like the discussion to continue in a meeting room. This is a very reasonable request and one that should be met in order to keep information about your child and family confidential.

Other health care professionals

You may meet other health care professionals with your child such as a GP or more specific specialists if your child has any underlying health issues. These professionals may also suggest that there are concerns around specific areas of your child's development, based on what you tell them and what they observe.

If a health care worker such as a health visitor or GP shares concerns about your child's development that you do not agree with it can come as quite a shock. You may feel tearful or angry initially. Ask them very clearly to state what their concerns are and why they have these concerns. Ask them also what the options are – for example, are they suggesting that your child needs further assessment or are they suggesting a 'wait and see' approach?

It is important that you give yourself some time to digest what has been said. Asking for a further appointment to discuss the issues can be a helpful strategy as it can give you some time to collect your thoughts and decide more clearly how you would like to proceed.

Professionals in an educational setting

Once your child enters an educational setting, be that a children's centre, a pre-school or a primary/secondary school, they will come into contact with a range of professionals who will be assessing their functioning.

If staff are concerned about your child they should inform you in order to initiate a discussion and find out your thoughts about this. Initially, the member of staff working most closely with your child will be responsible for assessment and should they have concerns they may request more specialist help. That specialist help may come from the SENCO who is based in the setting. You should be informed if there are concerns around your child and told exactly what these concerns are. Educational settings can request help from outside agencies during assessment if required, such as educational psychologists or learning support teachers.

If you do not share the concerns of school staff you need to make this clear. It may be that your child functions very differently at home than they do in school. Ask for a meeting with the person at the setting that you have been liaising with. Preparing for the meeting is key to helping you to feel calm and in control. Consider what you want to get out of the meeting: is your aim to get extra support for your child, for example, or is it to share with the staff why you feel your child's functioning is appropriate?

Write down a list of all of the questions that you want to ask and the points that you want to make. Ask the staff exactly what they think the problem is and what evidence they have of this difficulty. Be open and honest from the start and explain that you do not share their view but that you would like to hear what they have to say to identify a way forward. Further tips on how to handle these difficult meetings are coming up later in this chapter.

The other parent

Perhaps it is your child's other parent who has expressed a concern about some aspect of their functioning. This can be particularly difficult.

Tania says:

" *I'm worried about our son but John just won't listen to me. I know he's having problems at school. He's getting further and further behind each year. He struggles with his reading and writing; I suspect he has dyslexia. John just thinks he is a typical lazy boy and that he's not trying. John also blames the school; he says that the lessons are boring and this is why our son isn't doing well. It does cause a lot of arguments to be honest. It feels really difficult to be saying to my husband that this child that we've created together has a problem; it feels as if I'm criticizing him in some way too, which probably sounds ridiculous. The school have expressed concerns and at the moment I'm just saying that we are monitoring the situation and I feel stuck in the middle.* "

Sonia says:

" *Matt's dad and myself have recently split up; he's forever saying that Matt needs 'looking at', whatever that means! He thinks that Matt has problems but I think he is fine. I think that some of the reason that my ex is doing this is to get back at me to be honest. I'm not willing to accept that our son is having issues other than the normal difficulties that any child may face from time to time and particularly when their parents have just split up. I feel resentful that he dares to say that our son has problems, how dare he? I see Matt's flaws but I also see that he is a wonderful child who we are blessed to have. I think that this disagreement that we have about him has been one of the*

41

*contributory factors to us breaking up to be honest. I felt like
I was constantly battling with him not to have Matt taken to
the doctor. I do worry that now we are separated he will do it
without me knowing; I'm not even sure he can do that but it's
a worry.* **"**

Having different views about your child can be very upsetting. Both
parents love their child and both want to do whatever is best for the
child, yet when you can't agree on what is best it can be incredibly
frustrating and put a strain on the relationship.

It is important to focus the discussions on the issue rather than
making it personal and focusing it on your child's other parent.
Discuss the issue of the concern very broadly rather than looking at
it in terms of 'Should our child be assessed or not?'. This helps to
change the disagreement that you are having into a discussion. By
changing it into a discussion it becomes easier to listen to each other's
perspectives.

Ground rules during discussions can help to avoid conflict.
Listening is actually more important than talking when working on
developing an understanding of each other's views. When you are
interrupted it can be irritating and it shows a lack of respect for your
point of view. With this in mind you may wish to develop a ground
rule that involves you listening to each other with mutual respect.
Something may be said by your partner that you disagree with but
you can pick up on this once they have finished and it is your turn to
speak.

It is also important to check that you truly understand what your
partner is saying. Often arguments can occur when misunder-
standings take place. Once your partner has finished speaking sum
up what you think they have said and ask them whether you have
understood their point properly – is this what they meant to communicate to you? If not, allow them time to rephrase what they are
trying to say so that you understand them more fully. It is important
that you do really listen to what is being said to you rather than
focusing on what you are going to say when you get your turn. Your
partner has to feel that what they are saying is really being listened
to and heard.

Sometimes we make assumptions when we are in a relationship or predict what our partner is thinking and this can lead to conflict. Always check what your partner is thinking about your child rather than assuming that you know. Planning time to talk is important and not always easy. It is best if you can set aside some time to discuss your difference of opinion when you will not get interrupted and when no other family members are around. Speaking about issues like assessment can be stressful and these kinds of conversations are best avoided when you are tired or when you have been drinking alcohol. You should also never engage in these discussions around your child as this could be very damaging for their self-esteem.

If you find that you really cannot discuss your different opinions without arguing you could try writing down your points of view in a letter. This ensures that each parent's perspective is shared and that the information that you each want to get across is presented.

It is important to keep the issue in perspective and ask yourself whether it is worth ruining your relationship over. It may seem incredibly stressful right now but try to remember that this situation has occurred because you both dearly love your child and up to now have probably been in agreement with most aspects of parenting.

If you and your child's other parent are separated you may still experience the difficulties described and find that the issue of assessment and sharing concerns adds an additional pressure to a relationship that may already be fragile. Many of the tips offered in this section will still be useful whether or not you are in a relationship with each other. It can be helpful to expect that at times you will disagree, and to remember that it is the manner in which you deal with these disagreements that is important.

Relate offer free online relationship support and advice specifically around parenting at www.relateforparents.org.uk. The website includes a great deal of information and articles that aim to support parental relationships. There is also the facility to chat online to a Relate counsellor and a forum where you can post and access information and support from other parents. Alternatively, if things become very difficult you may wish to contact Relate and explore the option of couples' counselling in order to get your relationship back on track.

Relatives

It may be that one of your relatives has suggested to you that your child is not developing as they should. This can also be extremely difficult to deal with.

Joanne has four children and her mother-in-law is concerned about the youngest child's speech and language skills. Joanne says,

" *My mother-in-law is well-meaning and that is why it is so much more difficult to handle, I think. She keeps going on and on about how my youngest son isn't saying enough words for his age. She is forever going on the internet and looking up developmental stages and printing them off for me. I wouldn't mind but I have a qualification in childcare! Stan's speech is a little delayed but I don't feel that it warrants any further assessment but she just will not stop going on about it. Every time she sees him she will say, "Are you talking yet?" and I feel that she is building it up into a big issue. She also compares him with her daughter's child and I find that quite upsetting to be honest. Stan is an individual and he will do things in his own time.* "*

Joanne's mother-in-law is trying to be helpful but clearly her sharing her views is having the opposite effect. There is a very thin line between help from relatives and interference. It may be useful to avoid speaking about your child's development with them if you find that they then try to push an opinion on you that you find upsetting. Let relatives know very clearly that you have heard their concerns but that you do not wish to discuss them any further and that you will seek out their help and advice as and when appropriate.

It may be that you need to sit down and discuss their concerns with them to let them know very clearly that you have acknowledged them. This would also give you the chance to explain that you do not agree with them but to thank them for their concern or support. This can help to deal with the situation in a positive manner and avoid conflict if at all possible.

Acknowledgement and acceptance

There is a marked difference between acknowledging somebody's views about your child and accepting their views. Acknowledgement suggests that you have taken the time to listen to what they are saying and to explore the reasons why they have concerns around your child. To listen to their views is to acknowledge them and you can accept that these are their views without having to accept these views as your own.

Acknowledgement of views no matter how much they differ from your own demonstrates respect on your behalf. It is respectful to state that you are listening to that view even though it differs from your own. For example, Tom's mum has been called into school as staff are concerned about his behaviour. His mother has no concerns about his behaviour at home and feels that the meeting is unnecessary. Tom's teacher states her case about what his behaviour is like in school, saying, 'I'm concerned about Tom's behaviour; he is constantly in trouble in the playground and doesn't seem to be able to play co-operatively with the other children without lashing out or spoiling the game. The behaviour is getting worse and I want to look at monitoring this now and putting a behaviour management programme into place.'

Tom's mum can acknowledge what the teacher has said by saying, 'I acknowledge your concerns around Tom's behaviour. I, however, do not share your concerns as he frequently plays co-operatively with other children at Scouts and at home without difficulty.' This immediately makes the interaction friendly yet firm and states her point of view. Using the term, 'I acknowledge what you are saying' in these situations can be an extremely useful way of allowing the listener to realize that you do not share their point of view whilst putting it in a very polite manner.

It may be that you can see their point of view to an extent but do not fully share their concerns. It is useful to ask yourself whether you can share any of their concerns at all or whether you think that they are totally off the mark with what they are saying. If you can recognize where their concerns are coming from you can also acknowledge this.

Sarah tells us that her son's activity club leader shared concerns about his social communication skills when he was eight years old:

" *I've always known that Ben was a little what some would call 'odd' when it came to social skills. He has preferred solitary activities all of his life and can find social situations difficult. For example, Ben doesn't like noisy environments and hates going to birthday parties. He has some unusual interests for a child such as identifying flags from around the world – believe me, he knows them all, no matter how obscure they are! I recognized very early on that these could be signs of Asperger's syndrome as I am in fact a trained specialist teacher in the field of special educational needs. Ben is incredibly intelligent; I don't like saying that as I think it sounds conceited but it is true. He has a photographic memory and breezes through schoolwork. At the age of six he had completed the school's reading scheme. I thought long and hard about having Ben assessed for Asperger's and came to the decision that I wouldn't. I fail to see what a label would achieve to be honest. He wouldn't get any additional support and in fact he functions fairly well most of the time, having the odd meltdown when he is put into social situations. I also researched 'gifted' children and there are many traits of Asperger's syndrome present in the gifted child. I wondered whether Ben was gifted rather than anything else. I have been very keen to support his social skills as I recognized that this was an area that he needed to work on. This was how he ended up at an activity club where he could meet other children his own age and interact. One evening when I picked him up, the club leader asked if she could have a word. She asked me outright if Ben had a diagnosis of autism. It really shocked me to be honest, I think mainly because she was so blunt about it and I could feel myself getting very defensive and upset. I asked her why she was asking me this and she said that his social interaction skills were poor and that she works as a teaching assistant in a school and is experienced in working with children with autism and that Ben in her* *opinion fitted this profile. Keeping calm was difficult at the time as I wanted to hurl abuse at her, to be honest, for daring to speak about my son and compare him to others. All my motherly instincts kicked in at once and I wanted to grab him and run away. Instead, I told her that I acknowledged that Ben does have some differences in his social communication skills but that is because he is a very bright little boy who sometimes doesn't 'get' the activities that the average 8-year-old enjoys. I also thanked her for sharing her concerns and told her that if she wanted some advice on how to support Ben with his social skills I would be more than happy to sit down and chat with her about him. This incident did make me reflect on whether assessment was necessary if others were beginning to have concerns around his functioning. In my mind, however, I decided against it because if I had said to her that he did have a diagnosis, what would that have changed? He would still have the same issues that would need to be dealt with in the same way. Anyway, Ben is twelve years old now and I am so glad that I didn't have him diagnosed. He is much more sociable and has a group of close friends who he enjoys spending time with. His interests are now more age appropriate and he is very happy and settled, which is the main thing. I suspect the play leader thought that I was a parent in denial but actually I needed to trust my own instincts. What I'd say to other parents who are going through similar things at the moment is consider what you would get out of having your child assessed. If the answer is 'nothing' then I would question what the point of assessment would be. A label is something that lasts a lifetime; children grow and change.* **"**

Tips for hearing difficult news

We have already touched on some tips for how to handle the situation when somebody shares concerns around your child. It is particularly difficult to conduct yourself in a calm manner if you do not share these concerns.

Keeping calm

Firstly, remember that it is usual to feel a range of emotions when somebody is discussing your child in what you may perceive to be a negative manner. You may have heard of the fight or flight response. This is our body's inbuilt system of dealing with acute stress. It is a primitive instinct that prepares our bodies to either fight or flee in order to survive a perceived attack. The response is there to protect us from harm; it releases chemicals from our brain into our bodies to help us to either run away or fight the attacker. So if you feel like hitting the person who is telling you that they have concerns around your child, this is why! Or alternatively you may feel like getting up and leaving the room, which is where you can see the flight response being demonstrated.

It is helpful to know about the feelings that you experience firstly to normalize them and secondly in order to ensure you can remain in control during stressful situations. When the chemicals are released into our bloodstream, our bodies undergo some changes. Our breathing can speed up and our impulses quicken. There can even be an impact on vision with things appearing to be more sharply focused. When this instinct is activated we tend to perceive everything as a threat, and our rational mind fails to function. This means that when difficult news is shared with us we can overreact as we feel incredibly threatened. Our thinking becomes distorted and any fears and worries that we have can become exaggerated. Making clear choices while our bodies are in this mode is extremely difficult.

The fight or flight instinct was there to protect us from attacks from animals and so on when we lived in primitive times. In modern life we can rarely fight or flee the situations that arouse this response in us, so the response is rarely useful these days and can be counter-productive. It would not be a good idea to punch the health care professional who shares with you that they are concerned about your child's physical skills, for example. Neither would it be helpful to run out of a meeting with your child's teacher.

What is useful is to be aware of this response and to be aware of the signs that your body is going into fight or flight mode. You may experience physical symptoms first such as your heart rate increasing or your breathing getting faster. Or you may experience emotional symptoms first such as a feeling of anxiousness or tearfulness.

You will be pleased to know that there are a few benefits to your body going into fight or flight mode during times of difficult meetings. If properly harnessed, this mode can help to sharpen your thinking, which can be useful when putting over your point of view about your child's functioning. It can also assist you to be more decisive, which can also be helpful.

Breathing, as we have mentioned, is one of the first physical symptoms of anxiety and can lead to feelings of panic and loss of control. Concentrate on regulating your breathing if you are feeling upset as someone speaks about your child. Breathing in for the count of seven and out for the count of eleven is a useful strategy to help to regulate your breathing pattern. This technique also gives your mind something productive to focus on as it distracts you slightly from the situation while you count.

Keeping calm when somebody is talking about your child in a way that you disagree with can be extremely challenging. If you feel that you are about to lose your cool then we suggest that you take a break to think about what has been said. It is also useful to consider simply listening to the other person's point of view and thanking them for sharing that, then requesting a discussion at a later date once you have had time to digest the information.

Verbal communication

No matter whether you are liaising with a professional or a partner, verbal communication should always be respectful. Name-calling and swearing is undignified and unnecessary. Be very clear in what you are saying; write a script down beforehand if necessary to keep you on track.

Louise is a teacher and has to share concerns regularly about children's functioning:

" *I had to speak to a mum about my concerns around her child's functioning. It is never an easy job and she disagreed with me completely. I accept that sometimes parents and teachers won't share the same views but I like to work to find a middle ground* *for the sake of the child. This mum, however, started to be verbally aggressive towards me. She was extremely personal and told me that I'm useless at my job. I was mortified at the way she had spoken to me and felt threatened. I treat parents with respect and I expect to be treated with respect. I'm a mum myself and know how hard it is when somebody shares concerns around your child, I've been there too.* "

Be aware of the tone of your voice – using sarcasm during difficult interactions is not helpful. Raising your voice can be construed as becoming aggressive and won't help the situation.

Written information

Sometimes when we are stressed it is difficult to take in all of the information that we are being given. If a professional is expressing concerns around your child's functioning you could ask them to document this in a report. This will mean that you can read it and digest all of the information at your leisure. You should be clear, however, about who you are willing to allow the report to be circulated to – a section on consent regarding information sharing is covered further on in this chapter.

It is helpful if written material can clearly identify the specific concern with evidence for that concern. It is also useful if you ask for the professional to outline possible ways forward for you to consider.

Body language

It is important that you are aware of your body language during difficult conversations. While you may be saying everything appropriately verbally, your body language could be telling another story. If you are feeling defensive you are more likely to sit with your arms folded across you, giving the impression that you aren't engaging with the other person. Aim for body language that looks relaxed, even if you don't feel it inside. Keep your hands still and keep and maintain eye contact where possible. This will help you to feel more in control.

Second opinions

Consider whether it is worth asking for a second opinion about your child. You would need to think about who would offer this second opinion and, in actual fact, what you would do if their findings were the same as the professional who had concerns.

Consent

You should be asked to give consent to share information about your child between different agencies. This means that a school, for example, cannot share information about your child with any professional in the National Health Service without your consent.

If any reports about your child are produced you should ask who will be copied into these so that you are aware of where these records are being held. You do not have to give consent to information sharing between services, although it is usually in the interests of your child to do so.

Changing perspectives

It may be that right now you don't think that your child does need an assessment. Over time this may change, as Juliet tells us:

" Deep down I knew something wasn't right with Millie but I just thought she'd get better when she started school. Her behaviour was very challenging; she could be aggressive for no apparent reason. In fact, when she started school I was relieved to be getting a few hours off. I honestly thought it was just the terrible twos continuing at that point. Within a few weeks, however, I was called into school and the teacher expressed concerns about her functioning. To be honest I was quite rude to them and told them that she was a 'normal' little girl and that she just needed time to settle into the new routine. I came home and cried buckets full of tears. I asked for another meeting a few weeks down the line and it was the same story, she was behaving just the same at school as she does at home. The teacher broached having an assessment carried out on her and I immediately got defensive and

declined. A month on and things were no better. I could see that she was struggling to make friends, the other children avoided her and to be honest I understood why. I asked to meet the teacher again and agreed to an assessment. The assessment process is now underway. I suppose initially it was the wrong time for us to go through assessment as a family. It's still difficult now but I feel stronger as I've got the support of the school and that helps a great deal; I've apologized to the teacher since for being so defensive initially. But despite everything Millie is my baby and it was hard to sit with strangers and have them point out all her problems. "

Changing your mind about having your child assessed is fine. We all change our minds about things at times. Do not feel that just because you have decided against assessment at the moment it means that you can't revisit the idea at a later stage if you feel it would be useful for you and your child.

Monitoring

One way forward when others share concerns that you don't have is to agree to monitor your child's progress. Professionals could work alongside you and meet with you on a regular basis to feed back about your child's functioning in order to see if the difficulties that are perceived improve over time. If your child is in school and on the SEN register progress can be monitored via the use of Individual Education Plans, or IEPs as they are known. These set small, achievable targets to work on and progress is regularly reviewed.

You can carry out less formal monitoring at home by observing your child in different situations and noticing any new achievements. Some parents find it helpful to set their child small targets to develop new skills.

In summary

It is always difficult to acknowledge that your child may have difficulties in any area; when somebody else suggests this to you it can be even more challenging to acknowledge. This chapter has given you some practical ways to manage these difficult conversations more effectively. Ultimately as a parent you will want to do whatever is best for your child and sometimes this is not immediately apparent. Focusing on a child's difficulties can be distressing, so remember to focus on all the positives too and celebrate your child for being his/her unique self. Any decision that you do make around assessment will have been made based on careful consideration. You can assure yourself that you have made the right decision for your child at this moment in time based on the situation that you have found yourself in.

Chapter 4
Assessment

Once you have discussed your initial concerns with a professional, or a professional has indicated that they have concerns about your child, it may be decided that your child needs to be referred for assessment. There are many different things that a child may be assessed for and many different ways in which assessment can take place. There are also numerous professionals that you may meet during the assessment process. Some assessments may take place at home, others at a hospital or in a school setting. This chapter will help you to explore how best to prepare yourself and your child for the assessment process. You will also find out about other parents' experiences and read advice from professionals who carry out the assessments.

Information gathering

When you become aware that your child is going to be assessed it is important that you understand exactly what this process will involve and have some idea of timescales too. Assessment can often be a lengthy process; being aware of this right from the start can be helpful in understanding the procedures and will save you frustration.

Once the decision has been made to refer your child for assessment you need to very clearly understand how long it may take from the initial referral to receiving an appointment for assessment. Sometimes this can be a very lengthy process in itself. When you are referred, ask if the referrer knows how long it might take to get your appointment.

Waiting for assessment can be challenging. Once you have made the decision to move forwards you tend to want to get on with the assessment process as soon as possible. It is therefore helpful to know how long this period of waiting may last. Make sure that you have the contact details of the referrer so that you can chase up the referral if you have not received any confirmation that it has been received.

Do not be afraid of contacting the referrer to ask for an update on the referral and to ask for an estimate of the timescale involved before your child will be assessed. Referrals do occasionally go astray so you are quite within your rights to request confirmation that the referral is being processed.

Information online

The internet can be a useful tool for researching information relating to additional needs. It can also feed your anxiety and worries.

Sharon says:

" *My son was under assessment for difficulties with his vision. I took him to an assessment and the doctor started to talk about pressure behind the eye. I didn't really understand fully what he was telling me and I could feel my anxiety levels rising during the consultation. When I left I only remembered the odd word and looked these up on Google when I arrived home, desperate to make sense of what I was being told. The research on the internet kept leading me back to symptoms of brain tumours. Within an hour I was convinced that I'd been told that my son may have a brain tumour. Looking back, it was utterly ridiculous as this had never been suggested at all. I contacted the hospital in a real panic and discussed my fears with a consultant who reassured me that this was not at all what was suggested. I sometimes think that 'Googling' should carry a health warning for us parents.* "

If you do decide to use the internet to look at assessment for specific conditions then make sure that you access accurate information. Ask your consultant to write down the name of conditions that he mentions to you so you can be sure you are searching on the correct condition. Often early on in the assessment process you will not have the name of a specific condition and searching the internet may scare you as you stumble across 'worst case scenarios', so bear Sharon's advice in mind.

There are plenty of reliable sources of information on the internet and other parents can also give personal experiences, as in Roberta's case:

" *The worst thing that I found about the assessment process is the lack of information given. I went to my GP with concerns about my child's functioning; a referral was made for assessment yet I was then very unsure of the next step in the process. I ended up seeking support and information through my own online research. I used websites such as the National Autistic Society. I also found parenting sites helpful such as Netmums, which allows you to discuss issues and concerns with other parents. I accessed a lot of support and information too from our local ADHD/Autism Support group.* "

Look for advice from well-known organizations and national charities, sites like the NHS Direct website and Direct.gov to ensure that you are getting good online information. Start with Contact a Family, www.cafamily.org.uk, which offers excellent information on a wide range of conditions and can help you find condition-specific organizations.

Jean has a daughter who has undergone a great deal of assessment during her life. Sian is now nineteen years old and has complex needs. Her most recent assessment was a transition from children's to adult services. Jean recognizes the importance of information-gathering prior to assessment and says:

" *I find information now from a variety of sources. I have read books about transition and the COPE directory was useful when exploring options for my daughter once she left school. Over the years I have also built up a wide group of friends who are experts in additional needs and they provide me with a great source of information and advice. The internet has been a fantastic way of finding information and I use various parenting forums and websites as well as more local support groups. I am now confident at dealing with professionals and asking them for information. Make the professionals work for*

*their money and 'don't be afraid to ask' is the best advice that
I can give other parents around assessment.* **"**

When using the internet to find out information do use reputable sites
and remember that the internet is not regulated. Be aware of who has
produced the information that you are reading and for what purpose.
Some information that you will come across will not be applicable to
the UK.

Ask the professionals

Prior to assessment it is important to have the opportunity to ask questions in order to clarify the aims of assessment and explore what
exactly will happen. Knowing what the assessment process will
involve is key. It is important that you consider what it is that you
need to know in order to feel better equipped to cope.

You may wish to consider asking who will be involved in the
assessment. Some assessments involve a multi-disciplinary team of
professionals. If this is the case it is always helpful to know who
makes up this team and what their individual roles are. This can
lengthen the process but many parents find the extra information
invaluable. Make a note of the professionals' names and job titles so
that you can identify them more easily in the future. It is also worth
asking where each professional is based and for contact details. Just
because you may see a professional in school, for example, this does
not mean that they are based within the school and if you wish to
speak to them it is far easier to approach them directly than to leave
messages. Some assessments may involve just one professional, in
which case the previous suggestions still apply but will be much more
straightforward.

Once you know who is involved you need to explore exactly what
they are assessing and for what reason. Don't be afraid of asking
professionals whether they have any thoughts about what the possible
assessment outcome may be. They will obviously not be able to give
you a diagnosis prior to assessment but they should be willing to
discuss with you possible outcomes of the assessment. This can be
useful in helping you to prepare yourself for any diagnosis. Ask the

professionals how they will assess your child: will it be through observation or more formal assessments?

Sometimes parents are present at assessment and at other times this is not appropriate. Ask whether you will be able to be present during the assessment. If you can be present ask the professional whether they want you to sit quietly in the corner or whether they would like you to be actively involved in the process in any way. If it is not appropriate for you to be present make sure that you find out how the results will be fed back to you and when.

Find out how long the assessment will last and whether you need to do anything to prepare your child for the assessment. Do you need to bring anything with you such as school reports or specialist equipment?

Language around assessment can also be difficult to understand at times with abbreviations used frequently, such as CP for Cerebral Palsy or IEP to refer to an Individual Education Plan. If you don't know what abbreviations refer to in meetings it is important to ask. Never be embarrassed to say if a professional is using jargon or difficult abbreviations; professionals usually do this without realizing that what they are saying makes little sense to 'regular parents'! As you read material you may begin to identify abbreviations – make a note of them and then the next time you come across them you can use them to jog your memory.

It is also important to establish whether this is a one-off assessment or a series of assessments and to ask about the timescale that this will involve. The amount of time that assessment can take can be particularly difficult for families. Sarah says:

" *I had little information given from the professionals until they were nearly ready to diagnose. No one wanted to tell us that they were investigating for autism and it was very frustrating. The assessment process lasted about a year and a half, which was fairly quick compared to others but a year and a half is just too long, especially as most help won't be available until after diagnosis.* **"**

Anna agrees that the process can be a long one:

" Assessment was such a long process and that time delay had such a detrimental effect on my child. This was a period of huge stress for me, as initially I felt like I had to argue to get CAMHS (Child and Adolescent Mental Health Service) to take my concerns seriously. "

As in Anna's case, the length of assessment can clearly place a strain on parents and their children. Ask for a realistic timescale so that you are mentally prepared. Also question why it will take so long if the period of time seems unnecessarily prolonged. Consider the fact that a longer assessment period will mean that your child is given more time to develop skills and progress, which is a positive way of looking at it. Remaining positive is extremely important as it will help you to feel better about the process and will send positive messages also to your child.

Dr Louise Langman is a clinical psychologist. She tells us:

" Clinical psychology aims to reduce psychological distress and to enhance and promote the well-being of individuals, groups and society as a whole. Clinical psychologists have had a least seven years of training and research experience to enable them to help people to deal with a wide range of psychological difficulties, including anxiety, depression, relationship problems, learning disabilities, child and family problems and serious mental illness.

To assess a child, a clinical psychologist may undertake a clinical assessment using a variety of methods including psychological tests, interviews and direct observation of behaviour. "

She goes on to explain what to expect at assessment:

" It is likely that the clinical psychologist will want the parents, as well as the child, to fill out questionnaires or brief psychological tests to help get an understanding of the family setting. The psychologist will probably want to see the parents and the child together, then the child alone, and then the parents alone.

The psychologist may want to talk to the teacher, or even visit the school to observe the child in a different setting, or they may wish to talk to the child's paediatrician. They may want to do formal testing of intellect, achievement and emotional functioning. All of this will take time. The testing alone may take three or four hours, and the psychologist will probably divide that into two or three sessions to make sure the child is not fatigued, and also to have the opportunity to see the child on two separate occasions to look for any behaviour changes. Ultimately the psychologist will do a lot of listening and asking questions. This is good; you as parents want thoughtful suggestions and advice based on a thorough assessment, not a casual or sloppy approach. Try to be patient, but ask the psychologist questions as well as answering them. 🎵

Dr Langman's advice around assessment is, 'As both a clinical psychologist and mother, I would ask you to believe in yourself. You are the parent, and the expert on your family. Professionals are "hired help". Seeking support or therapy is not easy, particularly when you have a child with additional needs, but the benefits are worth it.'

Sharing information

It may be that your child is to be assessed by a health professional such as a speech and language therapist or a physiotherapist. If assessment is taking place outside of the school environment it is always a good idea to share this information with the school. Keeping the educational setting informed of any assessment is vital in supporting your child's development.

Sue is an early years teacher and tells us:

❝ *I often find that children come into school and are already under assessment at a child development unit, yet the parents do not share this information with us. This makes working in partnership incredibly challenging. Only recently I identified a child who I felt would benefit from assessment only to be told that he had been referred prior to attending school and that assessment was almost complete. The assessors had not been told that he was attending our setting either so it meant that they did not have a complete picture of the child's functioning. I think that parents may sometimes be worried about wasting a teacher's time. I would far rather that parents came to me to share such information so that I can support them through the assessment process as necessary. Conscientious teachers are always interested to hear about their pupils and parents should take every opportunity to discuss their children; if it is likely to be a lengthy discussion then ask for an appointment so that the teacher can give you the time and attention that you need.* "

Children sometimes function differently at home and at school. Make sure that you share the full picture with the teacher, providing them with background information leading up to assessment. Approaching the teacher to share information will show that you are an interested parent. If your child is attending an early years setting it is just as important to inform staff there about your concerns and any assessment that may be carried out.

If you take your child to school you could make a point of engaging in informal chat with the classroom staff on a regular basis. If your child is older or is transported into school a phone call or note to the school to keep them updated is key to maintaining effective communication. Developing a good relationship with educational settings is extremely important in the assessment process.

Parent consultation evenings provide the opportunity for you to meet with your child's class teacher and in secondary schools you may be able to meet with all the subject teachers. The time that you have with each member of staff is very limited so it is important to prepare your questions beforehand and plan what you wish to share with each member of staff. If you find that you do not have enough time to discuss concerns in detail ask for an additional appointment at a mutually convenient time. Do not feel that you must wait until the next parent consultation evening before sharing concerns or information; most educational settings operate an open-door policy whereby parents are welcome to call in to discuss their children.

You will find that if your child is formally assessed a report may be produced in time. Do check that a copy of this report has been received by your child's educational setting. If this hasn't happened request that a copy be sent to your child's named teacher in school and make sure that the report has been received by the school. If your child attends pre-school, nursery or a childminder's home it is also important that they have sight of any such information. It is highly important that settings are aware of any advice following assessment and any assessment outcomes.

You may be asked to give consent to share information about your child between health, education and social care services. It is important that consent is given so that staff working in each service are able to be told the information that they need to know about your child. For example, if your child is being assessed under the health service by a speech therapist, the therapist will not be able to share the outcome of the assessment with the school if you do not give consent. The school will then be unaware of the assessment or the work that they need to do with your child to support their speech development.

Common Assessment Framework (CAF)

The CAF is a shared assessment and planning framework that is now often used across children's services and local areas in England. Its aim is to help with early identification of children's additional needs and to provide a co-ordinated service to manage these needs. The CAF is used now as an approach to conducting assessment of a child's needs and establishing how these needs should be best met.

There are clearly identified stages in completing a common assessment and these include identifying needs, assessing the needs, delivering an intergrated service and reviewing progress. The CAF process identifies children's strengths as well as their additional needs. It takes a holistic approach and therefore you will find that you may be asked about a range of issues such as sleep, health care and family dynamics. Copies of the CAF form can be found online at www.education.gov.uk and you will see that it is quite a lengthy document. A pre-assessment checklist can also be viewed online and this may help you to establish whether a common assessment is necessary.

Any practitioner within the children and young people's workforce can offer you a CAF.

You are also entitled to request that the CAF process is undertaken if you feel that it is appropriate for your child. Likewise, a child or young person may request that a CAF is initiated for themselves. The CAF is a voluntary process and parental consent must be given. Some areas use the CAF as a referral tool. A Lead Professional is identified during this process and you should feel comfortable with the person who is chosen. You can nominate yourself to be the Lead Professional if you prefer.

Preparing your child for assessment

Once you have gathered the information and understand the assessment process you will be better placed to prepare your child for the assessment. How much preparation your child needs will depend on the age of your child and also on their understanding. Younger children may have little awareness of the fact that they are being assessed and many of the assessments are carried out through play.

Other children may need preparing for assessment particularly if they find strange environments and people difficult to cope with. Anna says:

“ *I had to prepare my son as it was a strange environment with people he didn't know. For the assessment process to be accurate this had to be carried out when I wasn't in the room with him. I have to say that information wasn't readily given to me around what the process would involve so I had to seek it out myself. The best I could do was to give him a rough idea of what would be happening and what the professionals would be doing.* ”

If your child finds changes in routine difficult it may be helpful for you to have a trial run to the building to show them where they will be going. You could also take photographs to remind them and talk to them about the assessment. If your child finds meeting strangers challenging you could request photographs of the professionals that you are going to meet so that you can share these with your child prior to assessment. Don't be afraid of making these requests – professionals will view this as a positive strategy to be using.

Helen's son has a visual impairment and had to go through medical procedures during assessment. She tells us:

❝ *I feel guilty at putting Harry through these assessments but know that it has to be done in order to obtain a diagnosis. I do, however, feel totally helpless and hate knowing that I am putting him in difficult situations. As parents we prepare Harry every step of the way through his assessments, for example, we give the equipment friendly names that he can relate to. The MRI scanner was a giant robot with little robots taking pictures of his body like an X-ray and the eye cameras looked like Wall-E so we would make reference to the film; other machines were Transformers. The professionals also helped to prepare him by using role play to show the equipment and explaining what the different implements are for.* **❞**

Sometimes you may be asked to leave the room while assessment is carried out. Dr Kairen Cullen, educational psychologist, explains further:

❝ *Some of the assessments that educational psychologists carry out with children are standardized and need to be administered in a low-key manner so that the child's performance isn't affected. I always explain what I do very carefully to the parents prior to assessment. I also explain the role of the educational psychologist and that I will observe the child in school as well as conduct more formal assessments. I work very closely with parents as part of the assessment process to formulate questions. I also make sure that the parents really understand the nature of my work and the assessment procedures. I think spending this time with parents to explain what I do is incredibly valuable and helps to ease any worries they may have. I also have a very flexible approach and if a child was very young or anxious I* *would review whether it was appropriate to let the parent sit in during the assessment process.* "

If you do need to leave the room you may wish to mention this to your child prior to assessment and explain to them that you will be waiting outside. This will offer them reassurance that as soon as the assessment is over they will see you. Depending on their understanding you may wish to also explain to them the reasons that you cannot be present.

It is useful not to begin to mention the assessment too soon to children who are anxious as this can give them time to feed their worries. You may wish to casually mention assessment a week before and then provide your child with more details on a daily basis. You could also have a word with people that your child looks up to, for example, a well-liked teaching assistant or sports coach, and ask them to mention the assessment in a positive manner too. Hearing that the assessment is going to be positive from someone other than yourself could reassure your child.

Dr Louise Langman offers advice to parents about preparing children for clinical psychology assessments:

" *Depending on the age and level of understanding of the child and the circumstances of the assessment, it may be recommended to prepare your child ahead of time for the assessment. Seek advice from the assessing psychologist on how best to do this. For some children anxiety may be elevated by too much advance notice of the assessment taking place, so speaking to your child on the day may be more suitable.*

Sometimes the psychologist may send a letter ahead of the assessment with a photograph of them on it to introduce themselves to you and your child. Sometimes the first meeting may happen at school with a teaching assistant present to support communication and familiarity.

Ultimately, reassuring your child that the person that they meet will be kind and friendly is important. You may wish to let them know that the person may ask them to draw some pictures, answer some questions about their favourite hobbies and so on. Your confidence and outlook about the meeting is important: if you are more relaxed and at ease about it, so will your child be.

The psychologist will likely thank the child for their participation and may give reward stickers or certificates to acknowledge their hard work. You may additionally praise them for being co-operative or brave, depending on the child's age and circumstances. 〃

Preparing yourself practically

In terms of preparation for parents the practical side is probably far easier than the emotional side. Assessment can feel like a helpless process for the parent; having practical things to do can not only help you to feel better organized but also give you something purposeful to do within the process.

You may find it helpful to buy a notebook that is specifically used to record your questions, thoughts and ideas around your child's assessment. It is very common for parental feedback to be used as part of the assessment process so you need to be able to provide professionals with information during meetings. Jotting things down with the date and time is a good way of developing informal records that may well be valuable for professionals during the assessment.

As previously discussed, assessment generally creates a great deal of paperwork and it is important that you develop a system for handling this. Gemma says, 'I learnt very early on to document and keep a record of everything and to back up any phone calls with an email or letter.'

Make a file specifically for your child and keep in this any documentation relating to appointments. You may be asked for dates of assessments as the process goes on and it is helpful to have this information recorded in one place. You can also develop a section in your file to record any communications that you have had with professionals. This will act as a reminder about who you have spoken to and when, and you can also review the information to ensure that professionals are carrying out the actions identified as necessary during the assessment process.

You may find that you are often asked for information relating to the pregnancy, birth and early life of your child. It can be helpful prior to assessment to think about any significant factors during this period and make a note of them to remind yourself. If factors during your pregnancy have relevance, you are able to request a copy of your maternity notes from the midwives or hospital. You may be requested to pay a fee for copying the notes.

Developmental milestones such as the age that your child crawled, walked and started to speak may also be asked about. Thinking about these milestones prior to assessment makes it easier to give accurate answers. You may have notes in the form of your child's 'red book' that was given to you at birth and updated regularly by your child's health visitor. This can form a useful tool for recalling developmental milestones. Routine health checks should have been carried out on your child from birth for the first three years or so. The health visitor is usually the key professional in identifying any potential difficulties that your child may have. If your child has seen any other specialist and you have their reports you should take them with you to your assessment.

Consider whether you have any documentation from an educational setting that may be useful, such as a school report or early years profile. If your child has an Individual Education Plan you should take that with you.

If you are not yet at the stage where you have any paperwork relating to your child's functioning that is also fine.

As a clinical psychologist, Dr Langman is highly experienced in working with families and offers the following pieces of advice:

" *Ascertain whether your child needs to attend the first appointment or not and plan your child care accordingly. Remember that the professionals will want to make you feel at ease. It is their job to facilitate you being able to share the information that they need. They are highly experienced in working with people who are feeling distressed and will most likely be easy to talk to. You may wish to bring a relative or friend to the meeting; let the professional know beforehand. You may find it helpful to jot down or collect information to take to the meeting. I would recommend making a note of any questions that you want to ask and taking these to the meeting. Also you can make notes during the meeting if you wish. And do ask questions in the meeting if there is anything that you do not understand. And finally make sure that you ask for the professional's contact details if you have any follow-up questions or comments that you need to add, or ensure a follow-up meeting is scheduled.* **"**

Preparing yourself emotionally

As we have read earlier, Helen's son's assessment for his visual difficulties requires medical procedures that can be uncomfortable. Helen tells us that she has to prepare herself emotionally for this:

" *I had to mentally prepare myself for some of Harry's procedures, which are not nice for my child and make him feel very uncomfortable. I soon realized though that some children are more robust and brave than their parents! The procedures were vital to him and so I knew that he had to go through with them. I made sure that I asked all the questions that I felt I needed to before, during and after, no matter how silly they seemed.* **"**

Talking to other parents who have been through similar experiences can be incredibly helpful to prepare you emotionally for assessment. It is also extremely important to hear that the feelings that you may be having are not unique to you, but that other parents have also felt this way. Claire is a member of a befriending group and she says:

" *Go to local support groups or meet with parents in similar situations. I truly believe that one of the best support systems freely available is the support from other parents. Realizing that I was not alone had a hugely positive emotional impact on me during assessment and I am still close friends with some of those parents that I met at this time. When my son was four years old I became a volunteer befriender in order to offer support to others.* **"**

You can find out more about befriending groups in Chapter 7.

Sometimes it is difficult to prepare yourself for assessment, particularly when it involves your child. You may have lots of feelings about the process, and sometimes writing down your feelings can be helpful. Some parents find keeping a diary during the assessment process is therapeutic. Writing down feelings can offer a release of emotion that is sometimes greatly needed. Diaries can also provide a way of documenting the experience and can then be reflected back on at a later stage.

Dr Langman suggests, 'If you are anxious about the meeting, plan a relaxing evening on the day before. If possible, visualize yourself meeting the person and talking about your child's needs calmly and thoroughly.'

Making assessment positive

It is important that the positives about assessment are considered as all too often the assessment process can seem a negative one for both parent and child. Many parents did share with us positive experiences and these should be celebrated.

Diana said:

❝ *We found the whole assessment process positive. We saw the same therapists and paediatrician throughout, which made a big difference to our son and us as we could build up a relationship with them and get to know them. We found the professionals positive in their manner even though our son was diagnosed with quite severe difficulties. The actual week of the assessment was great; the assessment team had a good model. We went and spent a week in a self-contained flat during the assessment and Lewis spent three hours a day in their developmental nursery. This meant that they got a full picture of his abilities. During that week he also went through all the other assessments with practitioners such as physiotherapists, speech therapists, clinical psychologists, educational psychologists and the paediatrician. At the end of the week there was a multidisciplinary meeting where we got the full, formal diagnosis of autism spectrum disorder, global developmental delay, hypotonia and hypermobile joints.* "

Developing a relationship with the professionals seems to be key in having a positive experience. Sometimes simply having your concerns listened to can be helpful as Louise tells us: 'The positive thing about assessment for me was that I felt like my concerns were finally being taken seriously and were being properly recognized and acknowledged.'

For some families the assessment process brought practical positives such as respite being offered. For others the experience allowed them to forge lasting friendships with families in a similar situation. 'Meeting the other families who had a child with the same condition was a wonderful source of support for us. They have been able to guide us, assist us with questions and support us along the way. I feel we have made some lifelong bonds,' says Esther.

It is also important to focus on what your child has achieved throughout the assessment rather than what they have not achieved. Chloe's son has a visual impairment and tells us:

" *At first I used to get myself worked up and see how many letters on the chart he hadn't been able to see. I had to give myself a good talking to and turn my mindset around. I knew for Jack's sake that I needed to be more positive about his abilities and actually celebrate what he could see. I now go into the assessments with a far more positive attitude. I know that he can't see all the letters, he has a visual impairment, but I praise him now for co-operating with the doctor and for tolerating the different tests, which at times are uncomfortable. I also build in a reward for him and we go for a treat as soon as we leave the building.* "

Children are very quick to pick up on their parents' feelings. If you have a positive approach to the assessment process your child is much more likely to be positive too. Rewarding your child for their efforts is extremely important. There are many different kinds of reward that you can use and emotional rewards are often the most valuable – for example, simply telling your child how proud of them you are or giving them a thumbs up sign and a smile as they enter the assessment room. Other rewards can involve giving a sticker, a small toy, a comic or a trip to the local cinema. Often, rewarding children with your time is the best gift that you can give them.

Make sure that you tell your child how pleased you are with them and point out exactly what it was that you were so proud of e.g., 'John, I love the way that you went into that room so calmly with the teacher,' or, 'Kim, you sat so quietly and really listened to that lady, I'm so proud of you for that.'

When relaying details of the assessment process to others remember to emphasize how well your child functioned and how pleased you are with them. Going into what is sometimes a strange environment and being assessed can be challenging for most children. Your child deserves a great deal of recognition for accepting the assessment process in a positive manner.

Sometimes it can be incredibly hard to remain positive about assessment particularly when things may seem so uncertain. Unfortunately, you cannot change the assessment process by worrying and therefore having a positive mindset is the best way to deal with it. Rachel Shaw is an advisory teacher and tells us:

** *Often there is a long period of waiting around assessment; parents may feel disheartened that it is taking so long for their child to be seen. I always encourage the parents to view this as a positive. Whilst the child is awaiting assessment they are developing their skills and maturing all the time. As a parent I appreciate that it must be a difficult time. Try to turn the negative into a positive by viewing the waiting period as a period where the child will be building on their skills.* **

Being positive is also extremely important to keep your child's self-esteem intact. Many children quickly feel discouraged if faced with tricky tasks and can rapidly lose interest in developing their skills. Children may also underestimate their own abilities if they are low in confidence. It is therefore important to praise and encourage your child, and to use positive emotion alongside the praise. Encouragement can be used before and during assessment and is expressed as an appreciation of your child's efforts.

As parents we are often our own worst critics, so you too need to make sure that you take time out to be positive about your own role in the assessment process. Reflect back on the things that you are doing well with your child. Give yourself a pat on the back for getting this far and getting your concerns about your child across so clearly at meetings.

In summary

Assessment can be a confusing time. Preparation is key so that you know exactly what the process will involve and how long it is likely to take. Being informed along the way is incredibly important so make sure that you ask for information from the professionals but also explore the value of parent support groups.

Remaining positive is vital not only for you but also for your child. Make time to think about all the things that your child can do rather than reflecting on their difficulties and give yourself credit for empowering yourself with information that will make the assessment process as straightforward as possible.

Chapter 5
Working in Partnership with Professionals

Being a parent is one of the most challenging roles that we ever undertake. Responsible parents make a commitment to their children for a lifetime and this relationship is of maximum importance to the child. Parenting is so much more than meeting physical needs like feeding, clothing and bathing a child. It also involves providing a safe and secure environment where children can nurture their abilities and achieve their full potential. Sometimes the role can feel overwhelming, particularly when difficulties arise.

Parents may feel fiercely protective of their children, something that is quite instinctive. From the moment that your child is born you learn everything about their personality, their mannerisms and their ways. Parents truly are experts in their own children and this needs to be fully acknowledged throughout the assessment process. As a parent it is essential that you realize your own importance in the assessment process.

This chapter will explore the importance of working in partnership with professionals to ensure that the assessment process is supportive and positive for all concerned. Working in partnership benefits not only you the parent but also the professionals and most importantly your child.

Supportive practitioners

When you begin the assessment process it can feel confusing and frightening. You may feel that you don't understand what is going to happen and when. Or you may feel confused about why professionals are working in a certain way, or what their aims are. It is important that you as parents are supported throughout this process so that you fully understand what is going on.

The amount of support that you require from a practitioner will vary from family to family. Some parents feel that they are coping well and that they require only a minimum amount of support as they have alternative support networks in place, for example, via parents' groups or family members. Other parents, however, find the assessment process very isolating and require a great deal of emotional support from practitioners.

Sharon is an advisory teacher who works closely with families, supporting them throughout assessment. She tells us:

" *I consider the most important part of my role as being supportive to families through the assessment process. I'm a parent of a child with an additional need myself and I acknowledge how isolating it can feel to be going through assessment. I hope that the parents who work alongside me would describe me as a supportive practitioner. I work very hard at building up relationships and trying to get to know the family. Some families seem to cope well without a great deal of support whereas other families feel that they need much more regular contact. What is important is that the family is aware that I am here to support them and I always say that there are no such things as stupid questions. A family really must ask any questions that they have, no matter how ridiculous they think they are. The fact of the matter is that if it is worrying you it needs to be discussed. I offer support in terms of information giving and signposting on to other services yet I feel it is the emotional support that I offer that is the most important aspect of my work. Parents do need professionals to ask how they are coping and to listen non-judgmentally as the parents share their feelings, worries and concerns.* "*

Sharon goes on to explain that empathy plays an important part in supporting parents:

" *Empathy is very different from sympathy; parents don't want sympathy. In my experience what they want is a practitioner who really hears what they are saying and takes time to listen. In order to support parents fully I need to be sure that what I am understanding from them is correct and sometimes this*

*means that I have to clarify information rather than assuming
that I have understood. If a professional has misunderstood
what you are trying to communicate then make sure that you
tell them; it is important that you have a mutual understanding
with your practitioner based on trust and respect for partnership work to be successful. We do get it wrong at times but only
know if you tell us.* **"**

Empathy is vitally important during the assessment process as an
empathic practitioner will help to make you feel valued and understood. This can help in reducing any feelings of isolation and
loneliness that you may be experiencing. When a professional shows
you empathy it also encourages a trusting relationship to form, which
is helpful when exploring issues around your child during assessment.

An empathic professional will support you in making the assessment process more manageable. You may find that during the process
you come across a number of different practitioners yet feel more
comfortable with one particular member of the team. This could be
because their manner and tone indicates that they are genuinely interested in what you say and you feel listened to. If this is the case then
make sure that you get their contact details so that you can keep in
touch with them for support throughout the process if appropriate.

Gina's child was assessed at the age of six and she recalls the
importance of receiving support from a caring professional. 'Having
a professional who was empathic made a huge difference. They took
time to explain what was happening and to not only find out about
my child but also to find out how I was coping and feeling.'

Clare also talks about empathy:

" *I think professionals need to be respectful of parents' views and
sensitive to the fact that coming to terms with having a special
needs child may be really difficult for some families. Some
families might never accept that. We were very lucky with our
assessment team. From the first instance they respected my
views as a parent and really took on board what I was saying.
They acknowledged what we were doing as parents to support
our child and gave us excellent advice on what else we could*

do to support him further. I also think that professionals having experience around additional needs is essential. One parenting course that I went on had a trainer delivering it with no knowledge of autism or severe learning difficulties. She said that she found it helpful to think of my child as an 18-month-old. He wasn't, he was a 6-year-old boy who in some ways might never have the natural reactions, particularly social ones, that an 18-month-old might have. I found it really disrespectful when she said that. If professionals have experience, particularly personal experience, they have a different level of understanding and empathy with parents. **"**

If professionals do say something that you find inappropriate or offensive regarding your child be sure to share this with them. You should be treated with respect throughout the assessment process and never be made to feel uncomfortable.

A two-way process

Developing partnership working is a two-way process that you as parents need to commit to alongside the professionals that you work with. It is important that you are honest and consistent with professionals during assessment. If you are finding the process emotionally challenging then you should explain this to them as soon as you feel comfortable in doing so. It is quite usual for parents to become emotional during assessment and professionals are used to dealing with a range of emotions from parents from hurt and confusion to anger and blame.

Simply stating, 'I'm finding this process difficult and feel upset today,' should be enough to ensure that professionals understand where you are emotionally. If you feel angry during the assessment then ask to leave the room for a few moments until you regain control of your emotions. No matter how you feel emotionally always remember that both you and the professionals are there to ensure that your child receives the correct level of support necessary so that they can meet their full potential.

Sharon, an advisory teacher, tells us:

" *Parents can experience a huge range of emotion during the journey through assessment. Professionals understand this and will try to be supportive. The best approach is to be honest about how you are feeling. Try to keep calm and if need be ask to leave the room while you gather your thoughts. A caring professional will show empathy for your situation; it does make it more challenging, however, when parents lose their temper. Sharing difficult news can be a challenge for professionals too and finding a way to do this, which is as least distressing for parents as possible is always my aim.* **"**

Hazel is a SENCO working at a school in Asia that follows the International Primary Curriculum. Hazel says:

" *Parents need to understand that professional educators want pupils to achieve and succeed to their full potential and as such parents need to communicate effectively with professionals. Parents have to have trust and this can only be gained by good rapport with the specialist teachers. If parents are unclear on how the processes work in educational settings, professionals need to make the process clear, explaining educational terms in user-friendly language. Parents need to know that teachers are approachable and understand their concerns.* **"**

If you feel uncomfortable working alongside a professional you could ask if there is an alternative member of staff who could take over your child's case. It is important that you work alongside practitioners who make you feel at ease, valued and respected.

Who's who?

One of the first challenges that you may come across is identifying who is involved in your child's assessment and what their roles are. A vast number of professionals may be involved, particularly if your child has complex needs, and this can become extremely confusing.

Set up a file for your child's assessment and include a contact sheet at the beginning. Whenever you meet a new professional ask for their name, title and contact details and ask what their involvement in the assessment process will be. Writing this information down will remind you later of who you have met and what their role involved. It may also be helpful to write down a little description of the person so that you can put a face to the name.

Sharon says that during her work she often gets mistaken for other professionals:

** It can get very confusing for parents when they meet a vast number of professionals during assessment. I use a business card now, which includes a photograph of me on it so that the parents can immediately remember who I am. In the past I've received phone calls from parents asking for medication because they thought that I was the consultant or asking for an exercise programme as I've been mistaken for the physiotherapist. Making a note of who you have met will help you to put a face to the professional, which makes it easier to contact them with any further questions that you may have. **

Once your child is in school a number of different professionals may become involved. These can include the following:

SENCO (Special Educational Needs Co-ordinator)
Every setting including pre-schools and nurseries will have a SENCO. It is their responsibility to work in partnership with you in order to identify any targets for your child and any intervention that may be required. They will also offer advice and support around assessment in order to ensure that your child meets their full potential. If your child has a learning need, you should be introduced to the SENCO, if this doesn't happen then ask who the SENCO is and request a meeting.

Teaching Assistant (TA)
May work with your child on individual targets as set by the class teacher, the SENCO or some other professional involved with your child. Many schools employ teaching assistants with particular skills in the area of special educational needs.

Learning support teachers

Usually employed by the local authority and may visit your child's school on a weekly basis to offer advice to the teachers around supporting children with special educational needs. Learning support teachers may work on a one-to-one basis with your child; they are likely to be based outside of school and therefore you should find out their contact details.

Educational Psychologists (EPs or Ed Psychs)

Employed by the local authority and can be requested to work with your child if there are concerns about his/her learning. An educational psychologist will support children or young people who are experiencing problems within an educational setting. The aim of educational psychology intervention is to enhance a child's learning and work can be done via assessment, in groups and by offering advice about strategies to adopt for both parents and professionals.

Class teacher/ pastoral teacher

Should be your first line of contact in school and they should have all the information regarding who is involved with your child.

Preparing for Meetings

When you receive your date for assessment or the initial meeting make sure that you are happy with the time slot given. If, for example, it is close to school pick-up time and you don't have anybody else to collect your child you aren't going to be able to focus on what is being said for fear of the meeting overrunning. Ask for an earlier appointment if necessary or see if any evening appointments are available if they suit your family better.

As mentioned in Chapter 2 you may frequently be asked for the history of your child's development to date. Having to constantly repeat this information can upset some parents so you may find it useful to have already thought about this and have documented it as outlined earlier. It is quite acceptable to explain to the professionals that repeating this information is upsetting and therefore you have prepared a synopsis of the information for them to read. You may also wish to request that a copy of this information is put on your child's file to avoid you being asked at future meetings.

Many parents worry that they don't know what to say or ask during initial assessment meetings. If you are asked for your views it is quite appropriate to be honest and to say that at the moment you are unsure of your thoughts on your child's assessment, yet you are open to the professionals' advice.

Active listening

Productive partnership meetings require both parties to engage in active listening. Active listening means that both parties really listen to the words that are spoken within the meeting and aim to understand the meaning behind them with as much accuracy as possible.

Sharon tells us:

&& *Active listening is so important in meetings and really helps to build partnerships. In my role as an advisory teacher I've been in a number of meetings where active listening has not happened and the outcomes are then not as pleasing for the family or the child. For example, I met with a family last week and the father refused to engage in the discussion and spent the time texting on his mobile phone. I find this disrespectful when I am trying my hardest to support them through what is obviously a very difficult time.* **&&**

When you go into meetings make sure that you are able to give your full attention. If possible turn off your mobile phone to ensure that you are not distracted by it.

If information is shared with you that you need to clarify then check your own understanding by rephrasing the information in your own words. So, for example, if you are told, 'Amy needs to undergo further assessment of her social communication skills using a multi-disciplinary approach,' you can clarify that you have understood this by stating, 'So what you are saying is that Amy needs to be assessed further now by the team we have seen here?'

Listening to information relating to your child can be difficult, after all, nobody knows your child better than you do. Give the professionals chance to speak, however, and don't be afraid of pauses in conversation – you do not necessarily need to fill these. Avoid interrupting the professionals when they are sharing information with you. If questions spring to mind while they are speaking make a note of them so that when they have finished you can ask them.

You should ask as many questions as is necessary for you to feel informed about what is happening. Open questions tend to elicit the best response for gaining information. An open question is one that doesn't receive a 'yes' or 'no' response. So, for example, rather than saying, 'Do you think that John may be dyslexic?' you could ask something like, 'What are the likely outcomes of John's assessment?' This gives the professional much more scope to explore all the possibilities with you. Also use the expertise of the professionals and ask them openly for their advice on the best way to proceed for your child.

Professionals may not always disclose to you what they are thinking about your child's assessment unless they are directly asked. Gail says, 'Almost every professional we came across was very tight lipped about what they were assessing for and we felt very alone and isolated. We were never given any advice and no one ever asked how we were doing.' Don't expect to be told what is happening; sometimes you may need to ask.

Don't presume that you have understood everything that has been said to you in the meeting. Clarify what you have heard in your own words; this will also allow the professional to check that they have given you all the information that you need. Likewise, professionals should demonstrate active listening skills during the meetings. It is extremely important that you feel heard and listened to. Practitioners should make you feel welcome and demonstrate to you that they are interested in what you are saying.

Recalling information

Often during meetings and assessment a vast amount of information can be shared. It is not uncommon to leave a meeting and struggle to remember what was discussed. Some parents find making notes in the meeting helpful. Unfortunately, however, while you are making notes you are most likely to have your head down concentrating on your written materials rather than be engaging with the professionals. This can compromise the relationship that you are working to establish and can also mean that you don't feel an active member of the discussions. One possible way to get around this, as mentioned earlier, is to ask a partner or friend to act as scribe and record any relevant information that you wish to remember. An alternative strategy would be to ask to record the meeting using a Dictaphone. This can be particularly helpful as it means that you can give the meeting your full attention without being under pressure to recall facts. It can also help if you need to relay information to the other parent or close family members. Sometimes as a parent the last thing you need when you get home from an assessment meeting is repetitively going through what was discussed. Having a recording of the session means that those who couldn't attend can hear exactly what was said rather than your interpretation of the facts.

You can also ask whether the outcome of the meeting will be published in the form of a letter or report and if so how long the circulation of this document is likely to take. Often documentation takes several weeks to collate and be signed off by the relevant parties.

Communication is key

Good communication is key in ensuring that parents and professionals work together in partnership. If something is said that you disagree with then you must explain this to the professionals. It is usual to have differing views on things and that does not mean that you cannot work together – differences of opinions, however, need broaching sensitively.

If a professional shares information about your child that you do not think is accurate you should say so in a calm and controlled way. For example, if the teacher tells you that your child's reading is not progressing yet you feel that significant progress is being made you should say something along the lines of, 'I'm surprised at that as at home I have found that she has started to read much more and also more complex material.' Remember that sometimes children function differently in different environments so it is important not to dismiss what is being told to you just because you have not seen evidence of it yourself. You could ask the professional to give an example to back up what they are saying and again this can be done in a non-confrontational and productive manner by saying something along the lines of, 'Can you give me an example of the difficulties that she is having with her reading in school, please?'

Jenny has a daughter who is twenty years old now and is highly experienced at meeting with professionals. Her advice is, 'Look at seating arrangements when you go into any meetings. My social worker gave me this tip and it really works. Try and get in between the clusters of specific groups or if it is a meeting where lots of professionals are coming together around a table make sure that you sit at the head of the table. After all, this is concerning your child and you primarily and you need to be able to remain the focus of attention. Be polite at all times but remain strong and remember you have equal right of communication alongside the professionals.'

Developing a relationship

Developing a relationship with the professionals involved with your child's assessment can take time. You should feel comfortable and relaxed when liaising with them. Share with them any information that you feel is important; the professionals can learn a great deal from you about your child.

Be honest and open with the professionals. If you are worried about the assessment outcome, share this information with them from the start. Ask the professionals if there is anything you can do to help your child at home. Professionals are there to offer you support and advice so you should use them as much as possible to support your child's functioning.

Jenny says her social worker went the extra mile to provide support:

“ Our transitional social worker has been an absolute gem. She has gone that extra mile to make sure that I'm looked after emotionally as a parent. She has even been able to get the local

authority to agree to a one-day transport service for my daughter to get her to her day facility so that I can continue with my college studies. She recognized when I was becoming stressed and depressed and signposted me to useful groups and individuals who could offer me the support that I needed at the time. She has gained an immense amount of job satisfaction from seeing how happy my daughter is now thanks to her supportive input. **"**

Complaints

If you feel that the professionals that are involved in your child's assessment are not working in partnership then you should make them aware of your concerns immediately. Often complaints occur as a result of a misunderstanding or poor communication and are easily resolved and addressed.

Initially speak directly to the professional that you have the complaint with and explain to them what it is that you are not happy about. Be clear in what you say and what you wish to change. Make sure that what you say is not personal and always remain polite. Jot down exactly what it is that you are unhappy about. You may find it useful to start the conversation using a phrase such as, 'I'm concerned that you said . . .'. This is a non-confrontational way of beginning the conversation. If you feel you can't speak directly to the professional then ask to speak to their line manager.

You may prefer to put a complaint in writing and there should be clear policies for complaint procedures at the school or health service that you are using.

Sometimes you may feel that you have too much on to face complaining. Gina shares with us:

" *I came across a number of pleasant but ineffective professionals; the term 'chocolate teapots' springs to mind. They did not know what to do or say and I felt ignored by them. I should have complained but at the time I did not have the energy to make the complaint. My self-esteem was rock at bottom and I felt that complaining would be pointless. We actually moved* *areas during the process. Initially we had a fantastic team yet when we moved we felt like we had dropped over the edge of the cliff as we received very poor support and help.* **"**

Carol made a complaint about her child's SENCO:

" *I had to put in a complaint about the SENCO as his statement was not being fully met. My advice would be to always follow the correct channels before getting to the formal complaint stage to see if it can be resolved. Don't be afraid to take the matter to the top level, the headteacher, and document everything. Make sure that your complaint is in writing with a time limit clearly stated by which time you would like a reply.* **"**

What next?

When working with professionals it is important that you understand who is doing what and when. Clarity of communication in meetings is vital to make the assessment process as straightforward as possible. Each meeting should ideally be concluded by a review of what the actions are going to be following the meeting and who will be responsible for carrying out these actions and by what deadline.

If this is not covered by the end of the meeting you should ask for clarification about what is going to happen next. Having a timescale to work to is important when you are undergoing assessment with your child. It will help you to make sense of the process and support you in understanding why at times there may be delays and it can feel like nothing is happening.

If timescales are given you can then chase up professionals if they haven't carried out the action as discussed. This is helpful in keeping track of what is happening around assessment and ensuring that professionals do carry out the work that they have committed to.

Also ask if there is anything that you need to do as part of the process or if there is anything that you can work on at home to help your child to develop their skills.

In summary

When you first have to meet professionals as part of the assessment process it can feel a daunting experience. As time goes by many parents feel more and more comfortable attending these kinds of meetings.

Always remember that you are the expert on your child and that you have a great deal of information to input into the assessment process. Organizing yourself prior to meetings is important so that you feel prepared, and asking questions is vital to ensure that you understand what is happening and what will happen next. If you feel that something about your child has been misunderstood or misinterpreted then do say so.

Chapter 6
Receiving Diagnosis News

Once your child has been assessed, you may get news that is difficult to hear. In this chapter you can learn about how to deal with difficult news. You will discover ways to discuss this with your child, their siblings, family and friends. Not everyone will take the news in the same way, and you will learn how to cope with this too.

The meeting

In the last chapter you read about how professionals can help and support you throughout the assessment process. Now read more about the actual meeting where you get the results of the assessment process, and how professionals can help you during this meeting.

It can make a big difference to you and your family if the news about your child's diagnosis is delivered in a helpful way, but this doesn't always happen. In interviews with 190 parents of children with profound needs, almost two-thirds were dissatisfied with the first information given. Doctors are typically the primary deliverers of news of a diagnosis, and have not always had training in communicating this in a manner that parents find helpful.

Most parents in the aforementioned study had been informed by a doctor and getting the news early on helped them, but sometimes medical professionals don't have the knowledge to be able to give you the clear answers you need early on as further assessment might be needed. When parents were told depended on their child's condition: parents of children where the cause of their disability was unknown were more likely to be told during or after the second year of the child's life, while parents of children with Down's syndrome were most likely to be told at birth.

There are things that professionals can do to help you during the meeting where they explain to you about your child's condition. Studies examining parental reactions to the 'informing interview' made the following recommendations:

✓ Both parents, in a two-parent family, should be together when told of their child's diagnosis
✓ Parents should be informed early on
✓ Simple, direct language without medical jargon should be used
✓ The informing professional should be both empathetic and supportive of the emotions you express
✓ Professionals should meet the parents in person
✓ Parents should be informed in a private setting
✓ Professionals should point out the child's strengths as well as limitations
✓ The way professionals talk should be tailored to the parents' needs for information
✓ If parents have a different cultural background to the professionals, this should be considered in relation to language interpretation, meaning assigned to the diagnosis, and potentially differing treatment preferences
✓ Nurses should evaluate the effectiveness of the informing interview in relation to the family's affective and information needs

Each of these considerations should be part of the process of an informing interview. Use the points above as a checklist and make sure that the professionals explaining to you and the setting your meeting is held in make the experience as positive as possible.

In another study, families of infants with Down syndrome and/or congenital heart disease were interviewed to identify the factors that influenced parents and caregivers' reactions to learning that their child had been diagnosed as having a chronic condition. Two-thirds of the times, parents had a positive experience, but families also reported negative reactions to outdated and inadequate information as well as to professionals who were insensitive to their needs. The study recommends that professionals need education to turn them into physicians who can sensitively and effectively 'break the news' to diverse families who have children with chronic conditions. It advises that doctors should PACE the news by:

✓ Planning the setting
✓ Assessing the family's background, knowledge and experience
✓ Choosing strategies that best fit the family's particular situation
✓ Evaluating the family's understanding of the information

Dealing with the diagnosis that your child is different

For most parents, being told that your child is different seems like bad news. Once you have had more time to live with your child's diagnosis you will feel the ups as well as the downs, but this can be little comfort in the early days. One study defines bad news to be, 'news that alters a person's view of the future: drastically and negatively'. Does that match up with how you felt on hearing news about your child's diagnosis for the first time? In a matter of seconds you have to get to grips with hundreds of ideas about how your child's future may be different to your expectations. Even if you have suspected there are issues, it is in this moment that you face them head-on.

Sue Atkins is the ITV *This Morning* parenting expert and author of *Parenting Made Easy – How to Raise Happy Children*. She outlines some of the more positive aspects to getting a diagnosis:

   The diagnosis is useful for getting the support or services your child needs and it is helpful in setting appropriate goals and gaining understanding that your child has a unique talent or unique need but I think it is worth pointing out that the diagnosis may come as shock or a relief to you and that whatever your reaction it is perfectly normal – some of you will have known from an early stage that your child was different, but for others of you it may be years before you guessed it and it may have taken you many visits to professionals to receive a clear diagnosis and for you to accept the new situation.

I remember I was teaching a Reception class when a little boy arrived on the first morning into the classroom and just ran round and round, and then he started eating the sand and rocking on his seat, sucking his thumb, looking bewildered and scared. His mum hadn't wanted to bring him to the two 'getting to meet the teacher' afternoons as she was frightened and scared herself about what was happening to her son but we helped the family get some professional help, support and a clear diagnosis of autism.

When I bumped into the little boy's dad one lunch time in the local butcher's he looked so relieved, relaxed and optimistic. I was pleased we had helped the family come to terms with something that was overwhelming and frightening. They were moving forward with their lives, facing the challenges and anxieties and getting the help and support they all needed. "

My child has a label

There are pluses and minuses to finally getting a diagnosis for your child. While uncertainty may be at an end, you may also suddenly feel that your child has a label. For some people, the diagnosis can be key to accessing the right services and support, but many parents feel that they have to continue to fight to get what their child needs. Naming your child's condition can help to explain it to others: if your child is seen as 'naughty', for example, it can be helpful to have a name for the condition that causes challenging behaviour. 'Sometimes you may feel that giving your child a label can limit them,' Sue Atkins says. 'Some parents will always focus on the difficulties and grieve their child's lost potential compared to others, but I challenge you to see beyond the diagnosis – to become a family who sees your child's challenges as making their triumphs even sweeter and your child's apparent "weaknesses" always being balanced by their amazing strengths.'

No news?

For some parents, assessment does not lead to a diagnosis. Some children have signs and symptoms that do not add up to an easily defined diagnosis. The meeting where you feel you will get all the answers can in fact simply leave you with questions. The experience can be very frustrating. Your doctor may struggle to give you a diagnosis because your child has a very rare condition, or one of a group of very similar conditions that are hard to differentiate. Some conditions do not fit into a specific disorder, while others vary in magnitude, or only develop as your child grows older. Even with the best medical care, there are some conditions that do not receive a name and diagnosis.

Although this can be distressing, according to the Early Support booklet, *Information for parents: When your child has no diagnosis,* treatment, therapy or teaching should be tailored to your child's needs, not to the name of their disorder.

If this uncertainty is affecting you and your child, contact Contact A Family (see page 101), or seek out specific organizations like Unique (http://www.rarechromo.org), which provides information and support to families and individuals affected by any rare chromosome disorder and to the professionals who work with them. There are also groups in most local areas for parents of children with a range of special needs: taking part in this sort of group does not depend on a diagnosis. To find out more, download the Early Support booklet, *Information for parents: When your child has no diagnosis* from https://www.education.gov.uk/publications/standard/publication Detail/Page1/ES16, write to DCSF Publications, PO Box 5050, Sherwood Park, Annesley, Nottingham NG15 0DJ, or phone 0845 602 2260 and quote ref: ES16.

How you feel

Sue Atkins says, 'After the initial shock of discovering your child is unique and special, gently and slowly change your focus from one of despair to gently and gradually starting to see it as an opportunity to learn how to help you and your child to explore and discover more about themselves.'

Atkins refers to the initial revelation of your child's diagnosis as a shock, and it is important as a parent that you remember this. However well prepared you feel you might be for the diagnosis, you will probably be stressed in advance of the meeting and your body may respond as if it has had a shock. Your body will release adrenaline into your bloodstream, which can make you feel:

✓ irritable
✓ tearful
✓ jumpy
✓ angry and/or confused

You might find it hard to concentrate as a result, and this can make it harder to understand what the consultant is telling you. You can cope with this by:

✓ noting down questions in advance of the consultation
✓ asking the consultant to explain in simple language
✓ taking notes
✓ recording the consultation
✓ asking for leaflets about the condition

Remember, it is fine to ask a professional to explain what they said. You might need to ask questions more than once, and review your recording, notes or leaflet several times after the meeting. It is quite normal to find it hard to take details of your child's diagnosis on board.

When you feel stressed, your hormones, including adrenaline and cortisol, are actually preparing you for emergency action: to fight or flee. In a meeting you are sitting down, trying to concentrate and communicate, and you lack any way to release the stress. If your child is with you at the meeting, you may feel that you need to keep it together for their sake. After the meeting it can be good to book in time to go for a walk or do something else physical. Ideally the same day, allow yourself time and space for physical relief – punch a pillow, go for a run. Ask someone else to sit with your child to allow you to do this. A physical release will help your body relax, and your mind may be better able to process the news about your child's diagnosis after a break.

Quick questionnaire: How do you cope with stress?

Different people respond to stress in different ways. Understand what happens to your body and it can help you deal with your response.

Watch next time you are under pressure. What happens?

Physical responses:

Do you
- ✓ become pale or flushed?
- ✓ get indigestion?
- ✓ have a dry mouth?
- ✓ need to use the toilet?
- ✓ shake?

Psychological responses:

Do you
- ✓ plan ahead in advance of a stressful event, imagining every detail?
- ✓ deny the event is happening?
- ✓ laugh about or ridicule something stressful?
- ✓ find out information and try to solve or fix the problem?
- ✓ get angry?
- ✓ get tearful?

More tips to help you cope

Although the professionals you are meeting with to discuss your child's diagnosis may be strangers to you, remember that they are probably used to breaking bad news to parents. Do not feel that you have to bottle everything up. It is OK to cry at the meeting, or explain how angry or upset you feel. Expressing your feelings can help you process them. If you feel too upset or angry to continue the discussion, ask for a break. You may want to step outside for a moment.

It can be hard to take on board news about your child's diagnosis and then move straight into making decisions about what to do next. Do ask for a further meeting if you think you may have more things to discuss, or you'd like to take time to process the news of your child's diagnosis before forming your views about the best way to help them. Never feel forced into making decisions: you can always ask for time to consider your options.

Sue Atkins says:

" *The reaction to hearing a diagnosis for the first time will be individual to you and how you react will depend on a number of factors such as:*

✓ *The severity of the diagnosis*
✓ *The nature of the diagnosis and the prognosis for your child*
✓ *Your child's age*
✓ *The presence of other associated disabilities*
✓ *Your previous experiences and knowledge of the condition diagnosed*
✓ *Your child's temperament*
✓ *Your own temperament*
✓ *The amount of help available*
✓ *How you were told about the diagnosis* "

An emotional journey

Your feelings will change in the weeks and months after hearing your child's diagnosis. You, your partner and other family members will go through a range of feelings, and you won't always be at the same stage at the same time, which can cause stress and conflict. Use this list to identify your own feelings.

How are you feeling?

✓ Confusion – why did this happen to us?
✓ Disbelief – it can't be true
✓ Grief
✓ Numbness – I can't take it on board

✓ Despair and feeling isolated
✓ Shock, questioning why it happened as it is so unfair
✓ Denial, refusing to believe this has happened
✓ Sadness and depression, feeling extremely low
✓ Feeling less isolated. Realizing others go through this too
✓ Beginning to feel informed and starting to cope
✓ Acknowledgement – knowing it will be OK
✓ Feeling calm. Knowing that you are doing well
✓ Happiness. Celebrating the positives

Read more about these feelings in Chapters 7 and 9.

Sue Atkins advises, 'It's perfectly normal to grieve after hearing a diagnosis and most parents experience a reaction similar to a feeling of bereavement – because while of course you love your child whether they have special needs or not, it is important to acknowledge that you have suffered the loss of a child who may have followed a customary path of development.'

It may seem that you are progressing forwards, feeling better about things, and then experience a day where you feel angry, frustrated or despairing. Our feelings are not always a neat and tidy progression, so don't give yourself further grief by feeling you are failing to deal with them: instead accept that everyone can have ups and downs, and being the parent of a child with additional needs can mean that you face a range of unexpected challenges. While experiencing ups and downs is normal, if you continue to feel distressed and hopeless, or feel that there is no way forward or that life is not worth it see your GP.

Different feelings

So far, we've mainly looked at your feelings, but your child's other parent, and the rest of the family, will be going through a range of emotions too. When you are upset it can be hard to be empathetic to someone else's distress, and this can lead to conflict, something that many parents of children with additional needs experience. Understanding that you and your partner have different feelings can help you deal with them. Go back to the *'how are you feeling?'* list and ask your partner to identify his or her feelings.

At times of crisis, it can be hard to help someone else when you feel you are not coping brilliantly yourself. That's why getting counselling can help. Ask at your meeting about support for parents to help you come to terms with your child's diagnosis. You can find out more about counselling in Chapters 7 and 9.

Tips to help you listen to your partner

Are you a good listener? We all think we listen, but a lot of the time we have our own thoughts and ideas taking up space in our heads, competing with what we're hearing. Life is busy, even more so when your child has additional needs, so it can be hard to really listen to your partner. Here are some tips to help you:

✓ Give your partner time to talk after the meeting
✓ Switch off your phone, the TV, and aim to ignore other interruptions
✓ Give your partner physical space, if this feels more helpful. Is it most comfortable to talk sitting across the kitchen table, in armchairs, on the sofa together?
✓ Look your partner in the eye if they are comfortable with this, but don't stare. Some people feel more comfortable sharing difficult issues without eye contact
✓ Sit still when you are listening, avoid fidgeting and breathe calmly
✓ Use a calm voice to talk: neither shout nor whisper
✓ Use non-verbal reassurance, like 'mmm' and 'ahh' to encourage your partner
✓ Reflect back what your partner says, for example, 'I can hear how worried you are about what's going to happen next'
✓ Let your partner finish what they are saying without interruption
✓ It is OK for there to be silence: you are creating space for your partner to speak
✓ Don't feel you have to 'solve' the problem your partner is raising. Often it is enough to say 'I understand there is a problem' – sharing can help your partner feel you are going to cope together
✓ Similarly, sometimes it is better to just listen than to debate a topic if you disagree

✓ Think about how you would like to be listened to, and acknowledge you and your partner may be different in the way you communicate

✓ Adapt your responses to reflect your partner's style of communication

If you and your partner find it hard to have calm communications, why not create a family communication charter e.g.:

✓ When another family member is speaking I will listen without interrupting even if I do not agree with what they are saying

✓ I will speak calmly even if I feel cross. I will use words to explain how I feel, not actions. For example, I will not storm out of a room, I will say, 'I'm feeling angry because . . .'

✓ I will listen to other people with respect

✓ We will turn off all mobile phones, TVs and any other distractions during discussions

✓ We will set a time limit on our discussions so that we are clear about how long they can go on for

✓ If I disagree with somebody else I will challenge their point of view sensitively and take responsibility for what I say

✓ We will all make a commitment to meet on a regular basis

Resources to help you and your partner

If you are feeling a strain on your relationship, here are some resources:

✓ Visit thecoupleconnection.net for online relationship advice, articles and a forum

✓ Use www.counselling-directory.org.uk/marriage.html to find a counsellor or psychotherapist specializing in couples' counselling

✓ Relate offers advice, relationship counselling, sex therapy, workshops, mediation, consultations and face-to-face support, by phone and through www.relate.org.uk

✓ Read *Special Needs Child: Maintaining Your Relationship* by Antonia Chitty and Victoria Dawson, which focuses on you, the parent, and how you can have a relationship that works.

Extended family and how to share news

Alongside talking to your partner, you will need to talk to other family members about your child's diagnosis. Some parents dread having to explain what they have discovered in the meeting, while for others it is a relief. Different people, and particularly different generations, can have preconceptions about certain conditions or disabilities. This means that family and friends will all react in different ways to what you tell them.

If you tell someone and they seem unsupportive, remember that they may simply be ill informed. While it can seem hard to have to be the one to deal with other people's emotions at a stressful time, most parents of a child with special needs find that they have to explain about their child's condition time and time again. Ask at the hospital for leaflets that you can ask people to read if you feel you are saying the same things over and over again. If you find discussing the subject upsetting, don't be afraid to say this and suggest that you need to continue the discussion another time.

It can be difficult to explain to your child's siblings about their sibling's condition. For younger children, you may want to work on a 'need to know' basis, rather than feeling you have to tell them everything at once. *Special Needs Child: Maintaining Your Relationship* has a chapter all about siblings of children with special needs and there is more about this in Chapter 9 too.

For any member of the extended family, though, the same message is important. Ask them not to rush to judge what will happen. As Sue Atkins says:

" *Of course, the presence of a child with special needs in your family alters your family relationships and the way it may now function, including the closeness of parents and other siblings. However, remember these changes may be positive as well as negative. It is down to your positive attitude and mindset about how you are going to handle this challenge.* **"**

Managing stress

Receiving difficult news is stressful, and the first step in dealing with the news is to accept that you will experience uncomfortable feelings. Give yourself some space to digest the news you have received. Here are some ideas to use on the day of the meeting and in the following weeks to help you manage stress:

Ideas to help you manage stress

Try to pick at least one idea from this list so you can make fifteen minutes a day for yourself. Looking after your own stress levels will help you help your child and your family.

✓ Walk round the block
✓ Work in the garden
✓ Take a bath with the door locked
✓ Read a book or magazine
✓ Have coffee with a friend

Another way to help manage your stress levels is to lower your expectations. If you are going through a difficult time around the time of your child's diagnosis, accept that your house may not always be tidy and not every meal will be home cooked. What can you do to make life slightly easier for yourself and diffuse stressful times of the day? Look at the times of day when you feel most stressed and see what you could change.

It can be easy to feel that you have to cope with everything on your own, and it might seem easier to keep to the family routine rather than let friends or family help out but it is important that you take breaks when they are available. If someone offers to look after the child(ren) accept – it may not be easy the first time and can seem like it's not worth the hassle, but with practice everyone will get used to it.

If you don't have any help available, try to break down the jobs that you have to do. Make a list – this can cut down some of the stress of keeping everything in your memory. Break down tasks into 'urgent' and 'important' categories, with a third section for things that are neither urgent nor important so could be done another day! Try to just do one task at a time: multitasking can become a habit, and it can make you feel that you are always juggling and under pressure.

Completing the urgent and important tasks on your list can help you relax once your jobs are done.

Another way to diffuse stress when coping with bad news is to remember the positives. This isn't about denying the difficult things, but instead about celebrating small achievements, for yourself as well as the children. Maybe everyone got out of the door in time this morning – give yourself a 'well done'. Remind yourself about between three to ten things that you are grateful for each morning or evening. Enjoy things like holding your child's hand, and try to stay in the moment rather than worrying ahead.

Another part of managing stress is to get as much sleep as you need or are able to. It isn't easy if you have ongoing disturbed nights, and children with additional needs often continue to have disturbed sleep well after you might have expected them to sleep through. As a parent, try to avoid caffeine in the afternoon/evening to ensure you can get to sleep. Read or watch something calming before bed, keep the TV out of the bedroom, and go to sleep at a sensible time particularly if you get disturbed nights.

If stress is causing you to experience insomnia, you might want help to learn to relax physically. See if you can find time to join a yoga or meditation class. Relaxing doesn't always come naturally and making time each week can help. If there isn't a class you can make, simply practice sitting and being aware of your breathing for a few minutes each day. Listen as you make your breath slower and deeper. If thoughts come into your head, simply be aware that they are there and let them move on while you focus back on your breathing. This can help you lower your stress levels.

In the long term your body can become used to living under constant stress, which can cause health problems ranging from headaches, constipation and stomach aches, to anxiety, which is caused by the same chemicals as your stress response. You might feel your heart beating faster, you might feel sick, or like you are short of breath. You may have a constant headache, or find that period pain worsens. Emotionally you may find it hard to concentrate, or you may be easily irritated, jumpy or tense. All this adds up so small problems can begin to seem unmanageable. If this sounds like you, take a few moments to do the breathing exercise in the paragraph above. Write down your worries, and accept that you may not be able to solve them all at once. Find someone to talk to: your GP can be a good starting point.

Alongside this, you might experience a panic attack: an acute feeling where you might shake, feel your heart racing and/or struggle to breathe. If you experience an attack like this it can seem very scary. In the long term, being under constant stress can lead to depression, a feeling that nothing good will ever happen. Whether you feel down and struggle to motivate yourself to carry on, or are in a constant state of anxiety or panic talk to your GP to get the help you need.

More ways to find help

Depending on your child's diagnosis and outlook, you may feel the need to talk to someone. Many charities and organizations run helplines, and sharing your fears with someone outside the family can be a real relief. The professional(s) who shared the news of your child's diagnosis with you is/are likely to have details of support groups nationally or locally. You might want to make a note to remind yourself to ask about this.

If you don't have any details of help and support, or if your child has a rare or unusual condition, try the Contact a Family (CAF) helpline. The helpline is free and provides confidential advice. Call 0808 808 3555 or email: helpline@cafamily.org.uk. You can get practical advice on:

✓ Benefits or tax credit issues
✓ Details of local parents' support groups
✓ Information about your child's condition
✓ Details of charities that give grants to families with disabled children
✓ Advice and information on any other aspect of caring for a disabled child

CAF also offer an SEN service, which offers advice on a broad range of issues related to special educational needs. The charity also has a Facebook page where you can post: www.facebook.com/contactafamily. Read more about help from CAF and other organizations in Chapter 7.

If you feel despairing about the news you have received or simply need a listening ear, you can call the Samaritans at any time of the day and night on: 08457 90 90 90 or visit www.samaritans.org. This help is available to anyone who is in any kind of distress. All calls are confidential, and while you can call about a specific issue, it is also fine to call if you just need to offload or share your fears.

Tips to help you deal with your child's diagnosis

Sue Atkins has some tips that you may find useful in the weeks and months ahead after receiving the news of a diagnosis:

✓ Give yourself time to come to terms and to develop an understanding of what this diagnosis means for you, your child and your family

✓ Avoid making any rash or major decisions in the weeks following the diagnosis

✓ If you need to, do seek another appointment with the professional who gave you the diagnosis so you can ask more questions

✓ Before any consultations decide what you want from the meeting and jot down any questions you have – it's very easy to forget them during a meeting. Don't forget to make a note of the answers. If you can't go to the meetings together do take a friend or relative if you want support and another pair of ears to help you remember what was said

✓ The diagnosis may affect each of you as parents differently – while one of you may be able to accept the diagnosis, the other may feel that it is not correct and continue searching for alternative explanations for your child's difficulty – that's why it's important to give yourself time and discuss all the decisions made about your child

✓ Be aware that there will be mixed reactions from your family and friends to the news of the diagnosis – some may be very supportive and some very hurtful and distressing

✓ Educate yourself about the condition that is affecting your child – use all the sources of information available to you – library, internet, other parents, organizations – knowledge is power

✓ Do seek a second opinion on the diagnosis if you feel the diagnosis you have received is flawed

✓ Get to know the professionals in your area – who are they? Where are they based? Do they work as a team or individually? Try to get to know the team that is dealing with your child and build a relationship with them

✓ Begin to keep notes of all your meetings with the professionals you are working with and if a professional is compiling a report on your child ask for a copy to keep with your records

✓ Many parents I've worked with find it very helpful and supportive to be involved with the organization or support group that represent children and families with similar special needs. I know making the initial contact can be a very big and frightening step but remember these groups can be a source of fantastic ongoing help and support. When you are ready, do make contact. You are not alone – and it helps to know that

In summary

Getting news about your child's diagnosis can bring all sorts of feelings into sharp focus. You and your partner can feel differently, which can add to the stress. Alongside confusing feelings, you will have to cope with making practical decisions, explaining to others what is going on, and the challenges of day to day life. Read Chapter 7 for more help with the practicalities following diagnosis.

Aim to make the most of any support available. At the appointment where you get news about your child's diagnosis remember to ask about support groups and counselling. Even if you don't get in touch straight away you may find a useful source of leaflets or support to help you explain to other family members and friends what is going on. Remember that you can ask for support at any stage.

Chapter 7
Emotions and Practicalities Following Diagnosis

Assessment and diagnosis can be a difficult time for families. Being aware of the emotions that you may go through can help some parents to normalize their feelings. Looking after yourself emotionally is important so that you can function to the best of your ability to support your child. Accessing support networks is also important as this can allow you to meet others in a similar situation to yourself while also accessing important information that you may otherwise have been unaware of.

This chapter will explore:

✓ Emotions that you may feel following diagnosis
✓ Fact-finding and where best to look for information around additional needs
✓ Different types of practical and emotional support available and how to access these
✓ Developing your organizational skills so that you feel equipped for any future meetings or assessment

Emotions around diagnosis

It is very difficult to predict how anybody will feel following assessment. Parents can experience a range of emotions from relief that there is finally a name for their child's condition through to anger or denial. Some parents may not receive a diagnosis when they would in fact have found a diagnosis useful and this too can lead to feelings of distress as they struggle to make sense of their child's needs.

In Chapter 6 we introduced some of the feelings you may experience around diagnosis. In this section we will look in more depth at some of the emotions experienced. You can also learn about 'coping mechanisms'. We all use coping mechanisms in order to deal with situations that impact on us throughout our lives. Coping mechanisms vary from person to person but may include being over-optimistic or perhaps becoming pessimistic. Other mechanisms may be anger or denial.

Throughout our research for this book parents consistently told us that there had been little emotional support available to them following diagnosis. Any emotional support that they had received was as a result of the parent being proactive and seeking out support. This is extremely concerning and was one of the primary motivators for putting this book together, to offer parents an outline of how they could prepare emotionally as well as practically for the journey through assessment.

Blame

Blame is a common reaction to diagnosis. You may blame yourself for something: perhaps you worry that your child's condition is due to a genetic disorder, or you may begin to scrutinize your pregnancy to see if there is anything that you could have done differently, which may have prevented your child's problems.

Ruth says:

" *I had some minor dental work done when I was pregnant with Sonny. I didn't realize I was pregnant at the time. When his difficulties came to light I blamed myself for having this done and was convinced I was to blame for his problems. It has taken me a long, long time to acknowledge that his difficulties were nothing to do with this.* **"**

Guilt

Parents are extremely good at feeling guilty. We feel guilty that we don't spend enough time with our children, that we don't have the finances to be able to buy them everything they want or to take them away as often as we would like. When it comes to diagnosis parents can feel guilty that their child has an additional need.

The five stages of grief

Some of the feelings that we have talked about in the previous section are outlined in what is known as the 'Five Stages of Grief' model. This model was developed by Elisabeth Kübler-Ross and was originally based on those facing terminal illness. It was however realized that the model can be applied to anyone experiencing a loss. When a child is diagnosed with an additional need parents can sometimes experience a sense of loss of what may have been had the difficulty not presented. For example, you may have dreamt of watching your child playing football, or seeing them take their first steps. Learning that your child has an additional need and may not ever be able to do these things can leave you experiencing strong emotions relating to this loss.

The model suggests that individuals do not have to go through each stage in chronological order or in fact even experience each stage. The reaction to the news that your child has an additional need will be completely unique to you but the framework of the model may be useful in understanding your reaction.

The stages are referred to by the acronym DABDA and these stand for:

✓ Denial
✓ Anger
✓ Bargaining
✓ Depression
✓ Acceptance

DENIAL

Some parents experience denial when given a diagnosis for their child. Denial can perhaps be useful to a certain extent, allowing parents to function throughout a difficult time. Denial can allow parents to believe that everything will be fine and give them hope that perhaps a cure for their child's condition will be found. It can also be helpful in reducing anxiety and anguish about the here and now.

Sarah says:

" *Looking back, yes I was in denial about Penny's diagnosis, she was two years old when she was diagnosed with cerebral palsy. I think at that moment in time though if I had taken on board the diagnosis and thought about what it actually meant then I'd have had a nervous breakdown. Being in denial allowed me to get up in a morning, to get dressed and to care for my family. It took time for me to begin to acknowledge Penny's diagnosis. I needed to come through the denial stage slowly and in my own time. I needed to make sense of the diagnosis by finding out more information. I also slipped back into denial at various points, particularly when Penny got her first wheelchair for instance. I could cope with using a buggy as that's what other children her age used at times but a wheelchair was a painful reminder of her difficulties. It was much more emotionally manageable at that time to pretend it wasn't happening and to think that it would only be a temporary measure as a cure would be found. I also thought that Penny looked more 'normal' in a buggy than a wheelchair and I kept her in the buggy as long as possible. I suppose it was my way of coping.* **"**

Sometimes denial can cause serious issues, for example, parents who are in denial may decline important intervention for their children. Usually, however, parents move through denial once they have had some time to adjust to the diagnosis.

ANGER
You may experience periods when you feel really angry about assessment and diagnosis. You may feel anger towards professionals who are working with you or towards your friends who have children without additional needs. You may even feel anger towards those who are dearest to you such as your partner or immediate family.

Accept and acknowledge that you feel angry rather than trying to deny it or squash it down: you'll find that your anger can burst out at inappropriate times if you do this. Talking about these feelings can help. Look for physical outlets for your anger – go for a run, shout out loud in the open air, or punch a pillow, for example.

BARGAINING

Bargaining refers to a stage that some parents may go through when they begin to acknowledge diagnosis but hope to somehow change the outcome. So an example of bargaining could be feelings such as, 'If I could just raise enough money for my daughter to swim with dolphins then I'm sure she would walk.' Bargaining may also involve faith and prayer, asking God to help your child to overcome their disability and promising that you will do whatever is required in return. Bargaining rarely provides a realistic solution.

DEPRESSION

At times depression can really take a grip particularly when dealing with the diagnosis of your child. You may feel worried about the future or you may not even be able to think at all about the future at this stage. If feelings of sadness or despair do take over your life you need to seek some medical help. Depression can be treated and you should not suffer in silence.

ACCEPTANCE

Acceptance is the final stage although we prefer the term 'acknowledgement' as after many discussions with parents it seems that it is difficult to ever truly 'accept' diagnosis but parents can reach 'acknowledgment' more easily. This is the stage where parents can acknowledge that the diagnosis has occurred and that life is going to be different to what was anticipated but actually it will have positives too.

Understanding your feelings

You may be able to relate to some or all of these feelings. It can be helpful to know about this model so that you can be aware of the emotional journey that you are on. You may also run through these feelings numerous times during your life in relation to your child's additional need.

Information finding

Many parents shared with us that they felt that they were given very little information following diagnosis. Some were given leaflets to take away and read but felt that they needed far more than this. In this section we will take a look at the different forms of information that are available and the pros and cons of each type of information. Sonia received her son's diagnosis in the form of a letter. She says, 'I'd have liked to have been giving a list of books or information to accompany the diagnosis. The paediatrician hasn't seen my son since diagnosis.'

The internet

The internet can be a useful source of information that is easily accessible. However, it can also lead parents to read information that may not be relevant or accurate. You must remember that the internet is not monitored and so you should always check the reliability of any information that you access online.

The internet can be a great way of tracking down resources to help with your child's disability, for example, more specialist clothing and nightwear. The other positive about the internet is that it operates twenty-four hours a day, seven days a week so it is always readily available.

Books

There are many different books available around different disabilities and additional needs. It is helpful to think whether there are any issues that you specifically want to learn more about so that you can narrow your search or whether you want a book to explain to you fully about your child's specific condition.

Ask the professionals involved with your child's assessment whether there are any books that they can recommend to you. There are a great number of books on issues such as behaviour management and educational issues.

Your local library will be able to help you search for appropriate books. If you look at www.amazon.co.uk you will be able to view a synopsis of the different materials available and read reviews that other parents have left.

Courses

Consider whether attending a training course or workshop would be helpful in developing your knowledge about your child's difficulties. You can ask at your child's school to see if they are aware of any parenting courses that are being delivered in the area. Your local family information service is also an excellent point of contact to find out more information about what is happening in your area. You should be able to find their contact details by contacting your local authority either via their switchboard or via their website.

Children's centres often have parenting workshops taking place on a regular basis and these can cover issues such as behaviour management and special educational needs. Your local Parent Partnership service may also be able to point you in the direction of suitable courses. Again, you can contact them via your local authority.

The benefit of attending courses is that you may meet other parents who are in similar situations to yourself. The courses are usually offered free of charge or at a significantly discounted rate. Some courses have crèche facilities, which can be useful if you have young children. Courses are often held in the week during the day, which can be difficult if you are working during this time.

If you are unsure about attending a course find out what the course aims and objectives are. This will help you to decide whether it may be of use. Also find out who is running the course and what their experience is, again this can be helpful in deciding whether or not it would be beneficial for you to attend.

Other parents

Parents who have a child with needs similar to your child can be a huge help as they often have a wealth of knowledge and information that you may not have come across. Parent support groups are an ideal way of meeting other parents and are dealt with later in this chapter.

Emotional support

Information searching can be useful in trying to make sense of diagnosis. Emotional support is, however, essential during this period. It is vital that you have some good support networks around you to share how you are feeling and so you can be listened to in a non-judgmental way. There are different kinds of support that you can access but you will often need to be proactive in finding it.

Anna says:

" *This is where the assessment process fails parents. There is emotional support out there but you have to find it yourself. Assessment can be an intensely emotional experience. Once I had found services such as a local support group I was able to access counselling. I would highly recommend that parents do seek out emotional support as you go through such a range of difficult emotions at times. Talking it through with someone really does help.* "

The type of support that you choose will depend on your individual circumstances but support available may include counselling, befriending services, support groups or friends and relatives.

Counselling

Counselling can be extremely useful as it can give you the opportunity to express your emotions in a safe and non-judgmental environment with someone who is trained at offering emotional support. You can attend counselling sessions either alone, as a couple or as a family.

Counselling will give you the opportunity to talk about how you are feeling and to explore any difficult feelings that you may be having. Counsellors will listen to you and help you to explore issues in order for you to develop better ways of living life. Counsellors do not offer advice but help you to gain a better insight into why you are feeling and behaving as you are. You could expect to attend weekly sessions for several weeks and it is important that if you are considering counselling you commit to this.

If you are considering attending counselling you may wish to consider whether you are going to attend alone, with a partner or as a family. You may be able to access counselling via your GP or a local voluntary organization. If you are employed you should find out whether your employer offers any counselling support; many larger employers do. Or alternatively you may wish to see a private counsellor, which will have a cost implication but ensures that you can find somebody who you feel comfortable speaking with. It may also ensure that you are seen more promptly.

It may be that getting out to see a counsellor is difficult due to the needs of your child. Some counsellors offer a telephone counselling service so it is worth asking about this if childcare is a barrier to you accessing support. There are also listening services such as the Samaritans, which may be a useful form of support.

Sometimes children or siblings may benefit from counselling following a diagnosis. Many schools now offer counselling services so if you feel that your child may benefit from counselling you could ask to see what is on offer. Again you may be able to access a referral via your GP or you could choose to find a private counsellor.

ChildLine offers a telephone counselling service to those under the age of eighteen and also offers advice to parents. The child does not need to give their name. The service allows them to just make a single call if they wish or to access a named counsellor on a regular basis if they prefer.

Lynn Wilshaw is an experienced Relate counsellor. She tells us:

" *When life is getting you down it really does help to talk. I work with people with a range of difficulties and who are experiencing a range of feelings and emotions. You need not work through difficult emotions around your child's diagnosis on your own. I work with both couples and individuals and counselling can help to understand emotions and also to understand relationships. If you find it hard to get out due to your caring commitments for your child then explore the option of telephone counselling. Sometimes telephone counselling can be easier at first if you are worried about meeting another professional. Make sure that before you book an appointment it is with someone that you feel comfortable with. Speak to the counsellor on the telephone, do they put you at ease? Can they answer your questions? Choosing the right counsellor is key for helping you to gain the emotional support that you require.* **"**

Befriending Schemes

Befriending schemes offer support through volunteers to parents of children with additional needs. Befriending services can provide important emotional support for parents and carers and can help in removing feelings of isolation that you may have around the time of assessment and diagnosis.

Lindsey Caplan, a service manager for Scope's north region, talks about the importance of their Face 2 Face scheme, which offers emotional support for families of disabled children.

" *I know that the service that Face 2 Face offers families is greatly valued by them, particularly those families that are going through diagnosis. This can be a very difficult time for parents and they may experience a huge range of emotions. The Face 2 Face scheme trains parents of disabled children to offer emotional support to other parents. This is crucial as it means that the parents truly understand what it is like to parent a child with an impairment. The training course that the parents undertake is comprehensive and ensures that they are confident at handling emotional issues. Our befrienders have continuous supervision from a qualified counsellor and child protection training. Many of the parents that are befriended go on to become trained befrienders themselves as they value the service so much.* **"**

Lindsey goes on to explain, 'Face 2 Face has schemes across the UK and we also offer an online service so even if there is not a scheme in your area you could access emotional support via email. We encourage dads to access our services and train as befrienders too; it is just as important that they get the emotional support that they need.' For details of your nearest Face 2 Face scheme log on to www.scope.org.uk.

National charities

There are a number of national charities that may be able to offer you support either in terms of providing you with information or putting you in touch with other parents in a similar situation to yourself.

Contact a Family is a UK charity that is an excellent resource for families of children with disabilities. You can visit their website at www.cafamily.org.uk and find a range of information relating to both health and education matters. They also have a national helpline, which is a freephone number and can be accessed for advice regarding any aspect of caring for a disabled child.

Contact a Family also run the SEN National Advice Service, which is a one-stop-shop service for special educational needs advice and information. They produce a range of publications and information about local events.

If your child has a specific diagnosis you may prefer to find a charity that focuses more specifically on one area of need such as ADDISS, which is the national Attention Deficit Disorder Information and Support Service.

Local support groups

There are a number of different ways that you can find out about support groups in your area. Ask when you are undergoing assessment whether professionals are aware of any groups that you may access. You can also contact your local family information service and parent partnership service. If your child attends school you can find out whether they have any parent support groups running; children's centres often run support groups too. If your child has a specific diagnosis, for example, of Down's syndrome or cerebral palsy, you may wish to contact a national charity that supports these conditions and ask about whether they are aware of any local support groups. Look out for local support groups in your local press and if you already know other parents in a similar situation to yourself ask them if they are aware of any groups that are running. Word of mouth is a good way of finding the right support group for you, and you can then find out what exactly the group can offer prior to deciding to attend.

Sarah says that she found parent support groups vital:

In terms of emotional support I think they are an excellent source of support and I'd advise any parent who has a child with an additional need to access their local group. One thing I will say though is that support groups vary. For example, the first support group that I attended was not right for me. It was very much about campaigning rather than emotional support. I didn't feel ready for that, I wanted somebody to hold my hand and tell me that it was going to be OK. 🟊

Louise now works for a charity supporting parents of families where a child has a diagnosis of autism and ADHD. Her own child has a diagnosis of autism, and she tells us:

🟊 *When James was diagnosed we were referred to the Early Bird course, which is run by the National Autistic Society. I would have liked the opportunity to attend a parent support group outside of Early Bird but there was nothing available in the area that we lived in at this time. I would have really liked some emotional support. The work that I do now provides this to families and I see what a difference it can make to meet other people who really understand what our life is like. I tried accessing support online via forums but it wasn't the same. I joined a group when my son was four and found it invaluable in terms of emotional support and advice.* 🟊

Other parents

Rachel's daughter was diagnosed with cerebral palsy and here she discusses how her health visitor helped her to access support from another parent in a similar situation:

🟊 *My daughter was diagnosed with additional needs when she was seven months old. Our health visitor at the time introduced me to another mum who had just been through diagnosis. I found this really helpful. Although we live in different towns, we keep in touch via email twenty years later. It is very useful to know other parents and carers who are in a similar position to yourself. Word of mouth is a really important tool; you can learn so much from other parents.* 🟊

Anna explains that you speak the same language at support groups and this in itself can be helpful:

" *I joined my local support group and found it invaluable as it allows you to talk to other parents in similar situations. Also having a disabled child means you can talk in 'code' a lot of the time using acronyms such as ASD, EP and IEP; you don't have to stop and explain who does what and what it all means as they understand.* "

Online support

Many parents use online forums to access both information and emotional support. There are many different parenting sites available and most have a special needs forum such as www.netmums.co.uk or www.mumsnet.com. There are also a number of sites set up for parents of children with additional needs such as www.parentsofdisabledchildren.co.uk.

As well as being used to access emotional support, these forums can be an excellent place to share information about any upcoming news or specialist equipment that may be about to be launched. Some sites also have a facility for buying and selling second-hand goods, as well as information about any grants that may be accessible to assist with funding specialist equipment.

Sarah tells us:

" *I do use parenting forums for support. I don't find them as useful as the face to face support that I get through support groups. They do have a place, however, and come in handy for asking quick questions or gaining support around specific appointments. I think that they are a good place to share information and I also like the fact that you can remain anonymous.* "

Louise says, 'Although I prefer to attend support groups I would encourage other parents to use the internet if you can't physically attend a group. Forums can be useful in terms of getting advice and information from other parents.'

Anna says that she has used forums on and off to gain emotional support for a range of issues relating to parenting her son. She tells us:

❝ *I would advise using forums as it is great to be able to talk to parents who are in a similar situation. The internet is twenty-four hours a day, seven days a week so you can vent on there if you need to at 3 a.m. Also it is often easier to write down your feelings rather than talking about them. I also like the fact that it is anonymous so this can make it easier to talk about the deepest fears that you may have.* **❞**

Key workers

Key workers are used to improve the services offered to families of disabled children and to provide a more coherent service for both the families and the professionals. The theory is that one named person acts to co-ordinate service input to the family from the range of services involved. Key workers may be employed by a variety of services and could be a family support worker, a teacher or a Health Visitor, for example. Parents may be able to choose to act as their own key worker if they prefer.

A key worker acts as a single point of reference for information for a family so that they can easily gain information as required. Key workers also support the family in identifying what their needs and the needs of their child are. Regular contact is maintained and support is planned in partnership with the family.

The key worker role can be a time consuming one and therefore it is essential that whoever takes on this role has the time to dedicate to it. Key workers are particularly important when a child has complex needs and there are more services involved with the family. These families should be prioritized for being allocated a key worker.

Our research suggests that parents are rarely offered the option of a key worker, yet where the option is offered it is a valued and useful resource.

Julie tells us:

❝ *We have a key worker for my son now that he is in secondary school and not only is it invaluable, I believe it is essential. It gives you the chance to build up a rapport with an individual member of staff who knows you and knows your child.*

Often the key worker can become your child's voice when you are not there. **"**

Dave found the model useful during assessment:

" *Everything was so new to us, I didn't really understand the roles of all the different professionals. Our key worker helped us to understand who was doing what and for what reason. We were able to build up a relationship with her and I didn't feel stupid asking her to explain things. She was also able to organize all of the meetings to fit in around my shift pattern so that I could be there; that's incredibly important to me. I think that all families should have access to a key worker during the assessment process as it is really helpful to have one point of contact to offer you not only the emotional support but also to be able to provide answers to any questions that you may have.* **"**

In contrast, June's daughter has complex needs and is nineteen years old, yet she did not have a key worker until she entered into adult services. June says:

" *The nearest people to key workers that we have had as a family have been social workers and the one to one support workers that my daughter had in school. However, the social workers had a huge caseload and sometimes were not able to get as involved as they may have liked to. My daughter now has a key worker at the day service that she is accessing and I have to say that it does make life much easier for me as I now have a focal point of passing on information.* **"**

If you feel that the key worker model would be helpful to you and your family ask a professional that is involved with your case if this is an option in your area.

Lead professionals

The role of lead professional was introduced by the government in 2005 in order to promote a more streamlined service. The lead professional takes on a co-ordination role like the key worker. Lead professionals' roles tend not to be as involved as key workers' and they act in a broader co-ordinating capacity. However, the role still involves offering information and emotional support. A family with a key worker will not need the support of a lead professional.

Organizational skills

Some people are, by nature, very organized, while others have to work a little harder in order to keep their affairs in order. The assessment process can result in various appointments, meetings with numerous professionals and large quantities of paperwork heading your way. It is helpful if you can develop good organizational skills early on in the process so that you feel more in control.

Many of the parents that we spoke to during our research for this book shared how challenging this aspect of assessment can be. One parent described it as 'a nightmare' and felt that she was more like a project manager than a carer.

By putting routines and systems in place you can develop organizational skills and manage the information that is given to you effectively. Checklists are a good way of organizing yourself. Many parents suggest that writing things down can be helpful to keep you on task and to remind you what needs to be done and when.

Vicky says:

“ *Each morning I make my 'to do' list for the day. Some of the things will relate to George and his assessment, such as chasing up the speech therapist for the latest report or booking him an appointment with the physiotherapist. Other jobs will be things like cleaning the house or going to the shops for some milk. I find writing it down is really helpful; it reminds me what I need to do and it is so easy to become forgetful when you are stressed. I also like crossing off the items once I've done them; it makes me feel like I've really achieved something. I look at the list each morning and prioritize what I need to do first. I often want to put off the jobs to do with George's assessment but I make sure that I deal with those first so that they are over and done with and I can put a big cross through them on my list. I also find that if I'm struggling to sleep at night I can write thoughts down on my list to deal with in the morning and it does help.* 🎔

Keeping a calendar or a diary is essential. You may find that you are asked to attend various different appointments. It is important that you write down when these appointments are as missing an appointment could result in your child's assessment being significantly delayed. It is also helpful to carry a diary with you that is up to date. This way, if you are asked for your available dates while attending meetings you are able to provide them straight away. Family wall planners are readily available from stationery shops and are a great way of compiling all of the family's activities for the week in one place. You can even make your own with one column for each family member or a specific column for appointments. You can then write on what each person is doing for every day of the week and at a glance you can be reminded of any important appointments that are coming up.

Preparation is the key to being organized. If you have an appointment booked for your child then make sure that you prepare for it the day before. Planning what you will wear and making sure that the items are out ready will help you to feel more organized and less stressed in the morning. Plan the time that you will be setting off for your appointment and make sure that you know where you are going. If you are travelling by car ensure that you have change for car parking. Often there are delays at appointments so pack a bag for your child with any items that they may need such as a change of clothes, books, toys or any snacks as appropriate.

Create a way of storing any paperwork that you receive so that it is easy to access. You may wish to use a box file, for example, and to simply put the most current document on the top of the pile so that they remain in chronological order. Or you could use a lever arch file and dividers to define where each report has come from if there are numerous agencies involved. The system that you create needs to work for you and be simple yet effective. Keeping documentation is extremely important as you may need to refer to it at a later stage. It is helpful if at the beginning of your file you keep a list of the names of all the professionals involved, their job titles and their contact details. This will help to remind you who does what and will provide you with an easy contact reference should you need it.

In summary

Assessment and diagnosis can be an emotionally difficult journey and finding the right kind of practical and emotional support can be extremely important for your well-being. This chapter has explored the different areas from which you may access this support. It appears that often sufficient emotional support is not offered to parents and you may need to be proactive in seeking out this support.

Information finding is also an important part of the process and you are going to want to find out as much as possible in order to support your child as effectively as you can. Always remember to ask professionals for recommended information and if there is something that you read that you do not understand make sure you ask for clarification. Support groups can be a great way of sharing information as well as meeting other parents in similar situations.

The amount of paperwork and the number of meetings that you may need to attend during the assessment process may feel daunting initially. Getting yourself into a good routine with managing the information is important to help you to feel in control. If you are feeling overwhelmed you could ask whether any of the professionals involved in the assessment could act as a key worker to co-ordinate services and assist you in managing information.

Chapter 8
Identifying Strengths and Formulating Strategies

In the last chapter we started to explore how to move on following diagnosis and discussed the importance of effective support mechanisms. In this chapter we will focus on identifying your child's strengths and how to develop these so that your child can meet their full potential. Behaviour management will also be explored in detail. We will also look towards the future and offer you support in beginning to plan more effectively.

This chapter will explore:

✓ Positive behaviour management strategies
✓ Celebrating your child's successes and planning the next achievable step
✓ Developing your child's skills through the use of interests and hobbies
✓ Identifying help that you may receive, including financial assistance
✓ Transition from children's to adult services
✓ Planning for adulthood

Positive behaviour management

Managing behaviour in a positive manner can be extremely difficult at times. If you take some time, however, to develop strategies you may find that other aspects of life can become easier. Parents are the most influential people over children's lives and behaviour. Many parents cited challenging behaviour as being one of the most stressful aspects of parenting their child, particularly when out and about in the local environment. John tells us:

" *Shannon will just throw herself to the ground if something is troubling her. Then if you try to get her up the screaming will start. We draw quite a crowd of spectators and that just makes the whole situation worse. I used to get really embarrassed about this and avoid going out with her but I've realized that I need to simply handle it differently. When she does this now I turn my back on her and wait until she has calmed down, then she gets up and we carry on with our journey. I've got used to the stares and tuts from passers-by. My top tip to other parents would be to try to stay calm on the outside even if on the inside you aren't feeling calm!* "

Using positive behaviour management strategies means that you draw attention to the behaviour that you do want to see. So if your child is being compliant you need to make sure that they are aware that you are pleased with this behaviour and be explicit about what aspect of the behaviour you particularly like. For example, saying, 'I like the way you are walking nicely holding my hand, that's really good,' makes it very clear what aspect of your child's behaviour is pleasing you and they will know to repeat this again in the future. Simply saying 'good girl' as you walk down the road may leave your child feeling confused about what aspect of their behaviour you are pleased about. At first it may be tricky to change the way that you comment on behaviour. If you are finding it difficult, use the phrase, 'I like the way that you are . . .' at the beginning of the sentence to help you to formulate specific praise appropriately.

Where possible you should ignore any behaviours that are not harmful or destructive. You may tell your child that you are ignoring the behaviour and you will engage with them when they are doing whatever it is you have asked them to do. Or you may simply ignore the behaviour completely and then when they stop immediately give them your attention. You will know the best approach to use with your child as you know them better than anyone else.

It is important to ensure that your child is clear about what you are asking them to do. Here are some tips to follow for giving instructions:

✓ Use your child's name to get their attention
✓ Make instructions short and to the point
✓ Give one instruction at a time
✓ Check that your child has heard and understood the instruction given. If you aren't sure ask them to repeat to you what you have asked them to do
✓ Allow time for your child to process the information
✓ Use picture cards to support their understanding if required (e.g. Makaton symbols or photographs)
✓ If your child doesn't follow the instruction they may need you to model to them what you are asking them to do, for example, you may need to show them how to wash their hands by washing your own hands if they haven't grasped that this is what you are asking them to do
✓ Avoid using sarcasm

Sometimes instructions can be too complex for children to follow or understand. Kat tells us:

❛❛ *I realized that I was overloading my son with instructions after attending a behaviour course. I was telling him to go upstairs, brush his teeth, find his coat, get his bag. He couldn't cope with that amount of information at once. I now give him one thing to do at a time and he functions far better and I feel much calmer too. It helps so much to break the information down into stages.* **❜❜**

Be aware that some children can be very literal in their understanding of language so make sure that whatever instructions you give are clear. Rachel is a behaviour expert and was called in to observe a child under assessment for Asperger's syndrome. She tells us:

" *The teacher was having great difficulty with the child's behaviour. I observed a PE lesson where the teacher told the class that they were to travel in a straight line moving forwards. This child was clearly engaged in the lesson and listening to the instruction. He travelled across the hall in a straight line and when he reached the door he opened it and left the room. The teacher saw this as him being defiant but actually he had a literal understanding of the instruction that he had been given and he was simply completing the task that he had been asked to undertake. It is very important that you are aware of children who may take instructions literally as this child was bemused as to why the teacher was unhappy with him when he had tried his best to do exactly as she had instructed.* **"**

Think carefully about what you say; instructions can often be misinterpreted, causing confusion for all concerned.

Keeping in control

Sometimes when we are faced with challenging behaviour we can find ourselves becoming extremely stressed and beginning to lose control. The flight or fight response that we are pre-programmed with can kick in when we find ourselves having to deal with our child's challenging behaviour. This can lead us to feel agitated, our breathing may speed up and we can lose control of our emotions.

Here are some tips to help you keep cool under pressure:

✓ Remember that the incident will pass
✓ Take some deep breaths, breathing in to the count of seven and out to the count of eleven.
✓ Think about your body language; we often clench our fists when stressed. Make your body language as open and non-confrontational as possible
✓ Lower the tone of your voice; we often find our voices rise when we are under pressure

✓ Avoid asking questions; give clear instructions in a calm manner
✓ Remember that for this situation to be resolved the first person that needs to calm down is you
✓ Model calm behaviour; if you shout your child may well shout back at you

Managing the behaviour

In order to manage challenging behaviour effectively it is important to try to find out what is causing the behaviour. Identifying a trigger for challenging behaviour can be difficult and there may be many reasons why a child displays certain behaviours. If you can identify the trigger or a number of potential triggers you are then better placed to try to avoid these where possible in the future.

Examples of triggers for challenging behaviour can include things like:

✓ Change in routine
✓ Hormones
✓ Sensory stimuli e.g. loud noises
✓ Lack of understanding
✓ Being told 'no'
✓ Tiredness
✓ Illness/pain
✓ Communication issues

It can be helpful to reflect back on episodes of challenging behaviour and to try to work out if anything happened immediately prior to the behaviour that can be identified as a trigger. Some parents find it helpful to keep a diary of the behaviour. These are often referred to as ABC charts and can help to identify possible triggers for the behaviour. If there is no trigger it may be that the child is being rewarded for the behaviour, for example, by being given attention.

Here is an example of an ABC chart:

Antecedent (what came before)	Behaviour	Consequence
There was a loud noise that made Charlie jump	Charlie lashed out and hit his brother	Charlie was removed from the room and taken upstairs to calm down

Here is a template that shows you how to complete your own record:

Antecedent (what came before)	Behaviour	Consequence
Write down here what happened before the behaviour. Include detail like where it occurred, when it occurred and who was there	Record the behaviour e.g. spitting, hitting, shouting etc.	Write down what happened just after the behaviour. What did the adults do? How was it resolved?

Consistency is key

When dealing with behaviour it is essential that it is dealt with consistently. You need to be clear, calm and consistent at all times, which can be easier said than done! Children feel secure when they know the rules and know that their behaviour will be dealt with in the same manner each time. If your child attends a school or a pre-school it is important that you communicate with staff there to find out how they deal with the behaviour and to see if there are strategies that they use that you could perhaps adopt.

It can be a good idea to utilize a home/school diary in order to share information between the settings. Use it to outline any difficulties that have arisen and note approaches used to help retain that consistent treatment.

Change can be extremely challenging and your child's behaviour may get worse before it improves once you put strategies to manage it in place. Children like routine and may therefore resist change: this is why consistency is so important.

It is important that, if another parent is involved with your child, you both adhere to the same rules. If you aren't consistent in your parenting your child will learn how to play you off against each other.

If you are concerned about your child's behaviour when you are out and about you can look at producing cards to hand out to anybody who makes comment or stares. Many parents carry pre-printed business cards that state that their child has an additional need and that challenging behaviour is part of their condition. Handing out one of these cards distracts the passer-by who will then focus their attention on the card rather than you. It may also help to educate people about the difficulties that some youngsters face with behaviour management and additional needs.

Rewards

The most effective way of reinforcing behaviour is through appropriate reward systems. We refer to 'appropriate' systems as often children with additional needs may be motivated by rewards that perhaps we may not have considered. Emma tells us, 'My daughter's reward is to sort out her pencils; it is a real treat for her to sort them by the colours of the rainbow and then once they are sorted to draw a rainbow. This beats any sticker that I could ever give her.' Rewards are only rewarding if they are motivating for the child. With this in mind it is worth spending some time considering what your child is interested in and how this can be used as a reward for positive behaviour.

Rewards do not have to be expensive or materialistic objects; they can come in many different forms and the most effective are often praise, hugs and smiles. Rewards should always be given immediately so that your child understands what you are rewarding. Initially your child should be rewarded each time they do something that you are working on with them and then reward less often as your child finds the task easier. When you do give your child a reward always make sure that they know why they are getting this reward. Tell them explicitly, 'Well done. I like the way that you are sharing your car with your brother.'

Use your child's name when you praise them so that they know that you are speaking to them and also so that they get used to hearing their name used in a positive manner. There are many things that you can praise your child for. These may include tidying up, sharing, helping, being calm and staying on task. Most children love to please adults and social rewards such as cuddles, claps or telling them 'well done' can be the most valuable reward a child can receive from you.

Rewards are important for grown-ups too. Don't forget to reward yourself; it is important that you celebrate the things that you are getting right. A simple 'well done' to yourself can make all the difference to the way that you feel.

Sanctions

Sometimes it will be necessary to correct your child's behaviour. Sanctions are strategies that you can plan so that you know how you will address any challenging behaviour. As mentioned, ignoring behaviour can be a powerful strategy to use. Children generally love attention and it often doesn't matter whether this attention is positive or negative. They would rather be shouted at than ignored. Rewarding positive behaviour and ignoring negative behaviour can be a good strategy to try. It is, however, important that you do reward positive behaviour; ignoring challenging behaviour without rewarding the good will just result in your child working even harder to attempt to get your attention.

Offering children 'time out' to calm down can also be effective if they are able to understand this strategy. Having 'time out' should not be seen as a punishment; it should be taught that it is a period of time when your child can calm down and compose themselves. Although there are many versions of 'time out' we prefer a positive approach and like to use 'the thinking chair'. This is an ordinary chair where the child can sit for a set period of time to calm down and to think about their actions. The theory behind it is the same as the 'naughty step' that many families use but it is a much more positive approach.

We all need time to calm down following an outburst of emotion. Teaching this to your child at a young age is important if they are able to process this information. Time out should always be timed and the timings should not be excessive. This is not a punishment, it is a mechanism to regain control. Sitting in 'time out' for lengthy periods is likely to make a child feel resentful and angry. It is a good idea if your child can monitor how long they have been in 'time out' by using a kitchen timer or sand timer to time the session. This also ensures that you don't forget about them and leave them sitting there for prolonged periods!

Removing privileges or loved items is another sanction that you may consider using. This works best for older children who understand the need to earn privileges. You may return the privilege once your child has complied or after a given amount of time. The privilege should, however, always be given back and ideally when it is taken away it should only be for a short period of time to have maximum impact.

Support around behaviour

Parents receive very little training around behaviour management. If you feel that you would benefit from some training it is often the case that you need to be proactive in finding training sources. Many parents found it helpful to discuss behaviour issues at parent support groups and to get support and advice from other parents. Kathy says:

" *I find that I ask other parents for advice, that way I don't feel judged. Other parents have some brilliant ideas about how to manage behaviour. I've done some parenting courses on behaviour but find that they don't fully understand what it's like having a child with an additional need. The ideas are OK in theory but in reality they aren't always possible to implement.* **"**

You may ask your child's school or your local children's centre for details about any behaviour management training that is happening in your area. Netmums is also a good source of information for parenting classes. You may find that your local authority has a Behaviour Support Service; they may also be able to offer you support and advice.

Boosting self-esteem

Self-esteem can be described as the view that you have of yourself. It is important that children have high self-esteem because it affects how they respond to others, their feelings and behaviour. High self-esteem generally leads to happier children. You can promote healthy self-esteem in your child and your input is key in making sure that their self-esteem remains intact.

Children with low self-esteem can be reluctant to try new or different activities. They may say that they 'can't' do things or speak about themselves in a negative manner, for example, labelling themselves as stupid. They may be over-critical of their own efforts and can give up easily or become quickly frustrated by tasks.

Children with high self-esteem are more likely to have a go at activities outside of their comfort zone. They will feel secure enough to make mistakes and then to learn from these. They may also be more willing to ask for help.

It is important to acknowledge the effort that your child makes. We have already spoken about the importance of praise; sometimes it is also important to praise the effort that has been put into a task. So if your child doesn't win the running race and finishes last but gave their all, it is important that this is seen as an achievement rather than a failure. Tell them how proud you are of their effort no matter what the result.

The way that you present yourself and speak about yourself can affect your child's self-esteem. If you tend to be a pessimist or harsh on yourself this will be picked up by your child. Listen to yourself speaking and consider whether you need to modify what you say in order to become a good role model for your child. By being positive you are providing a good role model to your child.

Life can seem challenging for children with additional needs and it is important that they are given time to reflect on what they are good at and what they are doing well. If your child is able to verbalize their strengths, encourage them to talk about what they are good at. Use the thumbs up sign to emphasize that you are pleased with your child if their understanding needs some signed support. Above all, believe in your child and focus on their strengths, whatever they may be.

Celebrating your child's success

It is very important to celebrate your child's successes. Professionals may be able to help you to identify your child's strengths and to build on these. Vicky Robinson, occupational therapist, tells us:

 Occupational therapy assessment identifies strengths as well as areas of need. It is important that we celebrate these strengths and build on them. Small achievable goals need to be set and should be based on the child's medium- and long-term goals. So, for example, a long term goal may be for a child to ride a bike; the smaller steps may be to work on balance, co-ordination, muscle strength and so on. Goals are frequently reviewed and evaluated to plot progress and fed back to the child and the parents. This is good for the child's self-esteem and rewards are used as appropriate such as certificates or reward charts. We use child-friendly outcomes measures in occupational therapy to plot progress. For example, we use a rating scale from one to ten with one being unable to do and ten being classed as being easy to achieve. Or we may use facial expression picture cards showing a sad face or a happy face. This is a good way of including the child in the evaluation process to ensure a child-centred approach.

Video is a good way of monitoring progress. When we see our children each day we may lose sight of their development. Recording them attempting different activities can help us to see the progress when we repeat the recording six months later and notice that they have achieved something that previously they were finding challenging. Children generally love to watch themselves on TV so this can also be a rewarding experience for your child.

Educational settings will be constantly reviewing your child's progress and setting small achievable targets. You should be kept informed regarding your child's progress and should be invited to meetings to review progress and celebrate your child's achievements.

Keep a journal for your own information and record the positive things that your child is achieving. Write down at least once a week three things that your child has done well. Reflecting back on this can be helpful to review your child's progress.

Promoting independence

Where possible it is important to promote your child's independence skills. Lydia says:

" *I am aware that sometimes I don't let Josh do things for himself that he can in fact do. It is easier sometimes to do them myself. For example, he knows where his shoes should go when he comes home from school but he often just leaves them in the middle of the hallway. It would be so easy just to move them myself but this isn't teaching him to become more independent. I now insist that he puts them away and I've noticed that it has now become part of his routine to tidy them up so we are working on hanging his coat up next. It is these little steps that perhaps other parents don't need to think about teaching their children that are so important in developing his independence skills for the future.* **"**

Establishing routines around independence skills is very important. Your child will find it much easier to develop and maintain new skills if they are practiced on a regular basis so that they eventually become habit. It is important to be realistic about your expectations and choose simple things that you know your child can achieve. Once you have decided on what tasks they can do you can think about how you can work with them to make sure that they are completed.

Some children like to use pictures to remind them what they are doing – these are often referred to as 'visual timetables'. A visual timetable is a way of showing using pictures, photographs or symbols what is going to happen during a period of time. The timetable should be placed where your child can see it easily and each picture should be removed once the task is complete. It is a good idea to put the jobs at the beginning of the timetable and to put a reward as the final activity on the timetable. For example, you may put a picture of shoes on the schedule to remind your child that they need to tidy their shoes away; you could then follow this with a picture of their coat to remind them that this also needs to be put away. The final picture could be of the TV, which shows them that once the tidying tasks are completed they will be able to watch TV.

You may need to break tasks down for your child and be very specific about what you would like them to do. For example, asking them simply to 'tidy up' may be confusing – they may need to be offered more structure such as 'put the DVDs back on the shelf, please'.

Interests and hobbies

Hobbies and interests are important for all children; they can be useful in building self-esteem and developing a child's character. There are many benefits to children developing interests and hobbies. Your child may have the opportunity to meet with other children and socialize with those who have similar needs and interests. This can be a great confidence boost and may help to develop attention, learning and physical skills.

When choosing a hobby it is important that you consider a number of issues:

✓ You should consider carefully what your child's interests and strengths are and how these can be used to identify a suitable hobby
✓ Financial implications may be something to consider. It is worth finding out how much the hobby may cost and whether this is feasible to fund
✓ You may also need to consider whether you have time to fit in a specific hobby; some hobbies can become very time consuming

✓ Would your child be suited to a home-based hobby or something that will encourage them to meet other children?

Many hobbies can be carried out at home – for example, doing jigsaws, computer activities or craft-type skills. Other hobbies may include joining an association or club. The Scouts, for example, have an inclusive approach and welcome children with additional needs to join their organization. There may also be specific clubs and activities on offer in your area for children with additional needs. Contact your local Family Information Support service via your local authority to find out whether any specific activities are on offer.

Claire's daughter attends a gymnastics club that has classes specifically for children with additional needs.

❝ *Beth joined the gymnastics club when she was around six years old and she has been a member there for the last five years. She loves attending and has met lots of friends. The teachers are fantastic with her and know how to get the best out of her. The club has helped her to develop her confidence, she even enters competitions now. I'm amazed at how co-ordinated she has become since starting gymnastics, it really has helped with her gross motor skills. Beth has won dozens of medals and I'm so proud of what she has achieved.* **❞**

Some interests can include the whole family. Megan tells us how her family enjoy geocaching:

❝ *Natalie has complex needs and sometimes it is quite a challenge for us to find an activity that we can all take part in. She has older brothers and I think they get frustrated sometimes that we can't always do things as a family. I had a friend who went geocaching and it sounded something that would suit my older boys yet at the same time something that Natalie could experience. Geocaching is basically an outdoor treasure hunt type game that is played all over the world. You have to try to locate the treasure; this is called a 'geocache'. This is done using GPS-enabled devices so we use our mobile phone. You* *can take the treasure from the geocache but you must replace it with treasure for the next player; there's a log book to complete too. You can log on to a website afterwards and share what you have found. It's a fantastic way of getting outdoors for a walk with a purpose. Natalie loves being outside and the boys love the thrill of finding the geocache.* "

For more details on geocaching visit the website at www.geocaching.com.

Other families find spectator sports are a good hobby to promote an interest and whole family involvement. Mike says:

" *I've always been a big football fan and have had a season ticket for my local football team since I was a child. Connor attends a special school and the football club donated some free tickets. Connor absolutely loved watching the match; he enjoyed the atmosphere, the music and the game. I had presumed he would have found it boring as he has learning difficulties and a short attention span but he actually was really interested in everything that was going on. I decided to get him a ticket the following season and there is a special part of the ground that disabled supporters can use. It's ideal as we know everybody who sits around us now and it is something that we can do as a whole family. Connor is football mad and insists on having the new kit and he's met a number of the players. I think it's fantastic that we are able to have this interest and hobby as a family.* "

Social care

Social care or social services as it was known is a statutory service within local authorities. Its role is to protect children from significant harm and to promote the well-being and safety of children who live at home or in the care system. Some authorities have a service manager who is responsible for services to children with disabilities or additional needs. These teams are usually referred to as the 'Children's Disability Team'.

Many people associate social care with child protection issues, but it is important to understand that this is just a part of a social worker's role. Social Care is also there to offer support and information that may be beneficial to your family. Often there is an eligibility criteria around whether you will gain support from a social worker.

Often families are referred to social care by a professional such as a paediatrician or health visitor. You can contact them yourself if you feel that your family may benefit from a referral. You will find their contact details on your local authority's website. If you don't meet the eligibility criteria you may be signposted to other local organizations that could offer you support. If you do meet the criteria you may find that you are contacted by a social worker who will carry out an assessment of your situation. Ask the social worker to explain to you how they will assess your family's needs.

The type of support that you may get will be dependent on the outcome of the assessment. Some families may get respite for their child or help within the home to support a child's complex needs. Support may be offered in the form of a nursery placement for a pre-school child. The support will very much depend on what services are available in the area that you live.

Respite care

You may be eligible for respite care for your child. Respite care is short-term care that may be provided for children with complex needs or for a family that is in crisis. There are usually different options of care available to support the family's needs. Sometimes there may be care for a couple of hours a week during the early evening where the child attends an activity club. Other alternatives may be where the child goes for a short break to a respite home or they may be linked with another family who provide support in their home either overnight or during the daytime. To find out if you are eligible for respite care for your child you should contact your social worker or your local Children's Disability Team.

Financial support

You may find that you are entitled to a number of benefits and tax credits as a result of your child's disability. Each benefit and tax credit has eligibility criteria requiring certain conditions in order for you to qualify. It may seem complex but there are a number of ways that you can gain support to help you to determine whether you are eligible for any financial support. Contact a Family's helpline is an excellent resource for information and confidential advice on any aspect of your child's disability. The helpline can also be contacted for advice and information around benefits. All advice is confidential and you can contact the helpline on 0808 808 3555. Alternatively you may prefer to email them at helpline@cafamily.org.uk.

Once you have identified which benefits you can claim it is important to do so straight away. It is often difficult to get benefits backdated. Your local Citizens Advice Bureau or welfare rights office can also assist you in identifying which benefits you may be entitled to and can explain to you how each benefit is paid. Some are paid directly into your bank account while others such as housing and council tax benefits are paid by your local authority.

Aids and equipment

Your child may require specific equipment in order to support their functioning. Some children, for example, require specialist seating or equipment to aid writing. Assessment should be made around any specialist equipment required. If, however, you feel that your child does require certain aids or adaptations that have not been provided you should discuss this with the professionals involved or your social worker if you have one.

Most health services have a designated continence service where you can get specialist advice and support around your child's toileting issues. Generally free pads are not provided until your child is four years old but you should check the policy in your area. Some areas also have a laundry service to assist with continence problems, again you should check with the continence service. You may also be eligible to have your water bills capped if you are on a water meter to help with cost of laundry.

Parent carer forums

Parent Carer forums exist throughout England and were set up through government funding from the 'Aiming High for Disabled Children' programme. The aim of the groups is to help families to get support and information when their child has an additional need. Many of the Parent Carer forums now have websites where you can access information about the service that they provide. They are often a useful source of local information and hold regular meetings where you can meet parents in a similar situation to yourself. Parent Carer forums also play an important role in influencing policy.

Advocacy services

You may wish to explore the possibility of using an advocacy service to support your child's point of view being heard. Advocacy services aim to protect the right of young people and support the right for their point of view to be listened to and considered appropriately. Advocates are trained to support children so that their views can be expressed about matters that impact on their lives. An advocate can help your child to understand their rights and the options that are available to them. They may offer your child support at meetings and make them aware of services that are available to support their needs. They can also support your child in making a complaint about services if necessary. Advocacy services vary across the country and are usually staffed by volunteers locally. If you are unaware of advocacy services in your area you can contact your local authority to find out whether they are aware of any appropriate services.

Parents as advocates

You are the most important advocate that your child can have. Sometimes it is not easy to speak up on behalf of your child and this may be a skill that you develop over time. Being well informed about your child's additional need is an excellent starting point. Asking questions is extremely important so don't be afraid to ask why things are being done and what alternative options there are for your child. Karen says:

❝ *I would never speak up for myself like I speak up for my son. I'm the sort of person who is always too shy to ask for help or support. When it comes down to my son's needs though I'm far more vocal. I realize that if I don't speak up for him then he won't have a voice. I am his voice and this gives me the strength that I need to be his advocate.* ❞

The future

It is important that you plan for your child's future and sometimes this can be a frightening thing to think about, particularly if your child's additional need means that they are highly dependent on you.

Wills and trusts

By setting up a trust and writing a will you are ensuring that your child's future is taken care of and that they will get support should anything happen to you. When you are thinking about writing a will there are many things that you need to consider and professional help is extremely important to ensure that the will is legally sound.

If you decide to find a solicitor it is important that you share with them that your child has additional needs. You may also wish to explore the option of setting up a trust fund for your child. This means that they wouldn't have to worry about managing money if something happened to you, as a trustee could manage the financial side of the arrangement. Mencap have produced a guide to setting up wills and trusts, which is well worth reading; you can download a copy from their website at www.mencap.org.uk.

Transition to adulthood

Compulsory schooling in the UK ends after Year 11. Many special schools provide education for children until the age of nineteen and at this point children will need to make the transition into adult services. This change can seem very frightening so it is important that you have an awareness about what may be involved even if it may be some time off yet for your child.

If your child has a statement of educational needs you will have annual reviews. When your child reaches Year 9 this review will be called 'a transition review' and is the beginning of the planning process. Your child will be invited to attend the review if appropriate and there may also be yourself, teaching staff, a careers advisor, a social worker or any other specialist involved with your child present. The review will be a chance to reflect on progress made over the last twelve months while also setting targets for the forthcoming year. A transition plan will be formulated by the school and updated each year, and you should always receive a copy of this plan.

You should begin to consider options for your child on leaving school as soon as possible. There are a number of factors that may influence your choice, including whether your child can travel independently, their level of cognitive ability and their personal strengths. You should also consider your child's care needs: Are they going to be able to live independently? Would you prefer for them to live in supported living accommodation? Or are you happy for them to remain at home with you? Also think about what interests your child – what are they motivated by? This can help to choose the right pathway for them in the future.

If your child can verbalize their wishes you should spend time talking to them about what they want for the future. Make sure that you get all the information that you need before making any decisions. Find out about all the different employment options and college options open to your child. When examining living arrangements be sure to look at everything on offer; even if you are fairly certain that you have a preference, try to keep an open mind. Careers advisory services vary across each local authority so you should contact your local service to ascertain what they are able to offer in terms of support for you and your child.

Once you have got the information that you need you should consider visiting different colleges or organizations to see which you feel would suit your child the best. Your child should also attend where possible.

You should ask about what kind of travel assistance is available for your child, if any. Your local authority will have a policy which outlines who is eligible for travel assistance and what the criteria for this is.

Looking after yourself

We are going to end this chapter by focusing on one of the most important things that you need to do for your child's sake and that is to look after yourself. As a parent the tendency is to put everybody's needs before your own but it is critically important that you take care of yourself so that you can then take care of your child to the best of your ability.

Consider for a moment what would happen if you were to become unwell. What would happen to your child? Caring for yourself is vitally important and something that should be a priority in your life.

If you are feeling under the weather or down it is important that you see your GP. You may need to highlight the fact that your child has recently undergone assessment and share any outcomes of this so that your doctor has a full picture of what is happening in your life. Stress can be an underlying factor in many cases of illness and this needs to be ruled out before further investigations take place.

Vicky tells us:

" *I always used to take pride in my appearance. Then when Corey went through assessment and we were told he had a special need I admit that I really let myself go. I stopped caring about how I looked and dressed; I put on weight. I felt really, really down not only about the situation but about myself. Over time I came to realize that I had lost some part of my own identity. The real me was proud of the way I looked and I needed to get this back. I joined a slimming club and shed some of the weight, not all of it I admit. I felt better though and then took pride in choosing some new clothes. I started to do my hair again and put on make-up. I looked better than I had in years and I felt better too. It gave my self-esteem a massive boost. I often hear parents, particularly mothers, saying that they don't* *have time to look after themselves; well I'd like to challenge that and say that looking after yourself is essential for your child's sake. If you feel down it's so much harder to go to those meetings, to face professionals, to be an advocate for your child. Investing time in yourself isn't selfish, it's an investment in your and your child's future.* "

We all need time away to recuperate, whether this is just a few minutes or an evening out with friends. While it is good to meet other parents in a similar situation to yourself it can also be fantastic to mix with people who have nothing to do with disability, to find friends who have similar interests to your own. Reece tells us:

" *I love playing golf; when I'm on the golf course I'm my own person. Nobody talks about my daughter's difficulties; some people I play with don't even know about them, which is nice in a way because I get to be the real 'me'. It gives me a release, an interest outside of disability and that is greatly needed at times.* "

Sonia has started studying in order to widen her social circle and also to give her an interest away from home:

" *When Charlie got diagnosed with cerebral palsy I'd expected to go back to work. I had a career mapped out in finance, a good job and qualifications. I didn't feel I could pursue any of this though as he needed me to look after him. It wasn't as clear cut as just sending him to nursery. He is often ill and needs a great deal of care and attention. I'll admit that I felt resentful at first; this wasn't the life that I had planned or chosen. After a while I'd become resigned to this being how life was going to be: I was a full-time carer. I still felt that I'd lost my identity though. Last year I decided to do something outside of the home for myself. I looked into various options and in the end decided on training to become a counsellor. I think that I've learned an awful lot about myself since Charlie's diagnosis and I've had time to think about emotional journeys that we take in our lives. Counselling would mean that I can give something back to others. I can work flexibly and be self-employed, which would suit me as I can work around Charlie's needs. It will also give me back my identity, my feeling of self-worth. I'm so glad that I enrolled on the course. I have met people from a range of backgrounds and I get the chance to be the real me when I'm at college. I can be seen as being 'Sonia' rather than 'Charlie's mum' and while I love being a mum it is really important to me that I have my own identity too.* "

Mixing with people outside of the world of disability can be challenging yet is also essential in order to keep perspective of the problems that you face. Deanne says:

" *None of my friends have children with special needs and they don't understand how difficult it can be for me to, for example, arrange a babysitter for a night out. I'm a single mum and Star is tube fed; her needs are significant and I can't just decide at the drop of a hat that I'm going out like they often can. What I do love about having these girls as friends though is that they don't talk about disability. It gives me an outlet, some normality. I do get frustrated at times that they don't understand how difficult life can be but I also have great fun when I'm with them and I always feel so much better after making the effort to go out, even if it does take great organization in order to achieve a few hours at the pub!* "

As parents we can often be harsh on ourselves about the things that we perceive that we have got wrong around parenting. It is, however, incredibly important that we celebrate all the things that we have succeeded at. Parenting is a difficult job and even more challenging when a child has an additional need. Take some time to reflect on the things that you have achieved as a parent that you are proud of; there will be many when you sit down and think about it.

We all have limitations and there may be periods in your life when you feel that you aren't coping or there may be situations that you find particularly challenging. Don't let these periods overshadow all the fantastic things that you are achieving; it is important that you keep them in perspective. If you need help or advice make sure that you ask for it. If you don't feel that you can ask a professional seek guidance from a parenting organization; you don't have to cope by yourself.

Eating and sleeping well are important not only for your physical health but also for your emotional well-being. If you are grabbing snacks constantly or eating your child's leftovers you need to address your eating habits. You must make time to eat proper nutritious meals if you are going to be equipped to support your child to the best of your ability. Sleeping is also important and can be a challenge if your child has sleep issues. You may need to explore respite options or sleep during the day if possible while your child is at school. If you are sleep-deprived you will be unable to function, which can impact on every aspect of your life.

It is not always possible to have time away from the home in order to gain some relaxation space. It is, however, essential that you build in at least fifteen minutes a day of time for yourself. This can be time that you can look forward to, during which you engage in something that you find relaxing. You may need to plan this time for when your child is in bed or out of the home environment. Relaxation activities can be as simple as reading a magazine, having a quiet cup of tea, gardening or telephoning a friend. These activities are vital in order to keep you mentally and emotionally well and will help you to recharge your batteries.

In summary

In this chapter we have covered a wide range of subjects to help you to move on from diagnosis and plan positive strategies to support your child's development. There may be organizations that you need to contact as a result of your reading, or ideas that you need to take time to consider, for example, thinking about what sort of hobby might be suitable for your child.

The key message in this chapter is not to forget the importance of looking after yourself. It is important that you look after yourself in order to look after your child to the best of your ability. Spending time on recreational activities is an investment in your own personal well-being and you should not feel guilty for having time away from your child. Parenting is a challenging role and in order to enjoy it you also need time to reaffirm your own identify and to be a person in your own right.

Chapter 9
Moving On from Diagnosis

Parents can feel a huge range of emotions following diagnosis. The initial shock and disbelief that this is happening can then move on to blame and guilt. Eventually most parents will overcome this stage and be ready to move on from diagnosis.

This chapter will explore:

✓ The importance of communication in helping you to move on
✓ Supporting other members of your family through diagnosis and helping them to move on
✓ Managing your stress levels so that you can look after your child more effectively
✓ Enjoying your child and exploring how to make the diagnosis in some way positive
✓ Addressing any difficulties within the education system

Communication is key

Communicating how you feel is extremely important in helping you to move on from the diagnosis that your child has received. There is no right or wrong way to experience the emotions that you have felt about assessment and diagnosis; we are all individuals and experience them in our own way. How you experience these feelings will depend on your personality and your own personal coping style.

Some parents report that they feel a sense of relief immediately following diagnosis and they continue to feel better each day. Others report feeling down for long periods of time. It is important that you allow yourself time to experience these emotions and that you are patient with yourself.

Dave recalls:

❝ *I felt so shocked, even though I knew that there was something not quite right to hear it given a name was incredibly shocking. It was as though nobody could understand how I was feeling at that moment. I was angry because the world was carrying on regardless and here I was hearing this news that shattered my world. I then felt incredibly down as if I was falling into a deep, deep, dark hole with no light at the end of the tunnel. Those days following diagnosis were the worst that I've ever experienced in my life but I'm pleased to say that things do get better.* **"**

In contrast, Paula explains how she felt a sense of relief:

" *Nobody wants to hear that their child has an additional need but when I received the diagnosis I felt myself suddenly relax for the first time in months. It was like a burden had been lifted in a way. I could stop the fight now to find out what was the matter. I had a label, a reason for why my child was functioning in a different way. It also helped me because I could take some of that blame away from myself. It wasn't my fault if my child couldn't stand in a queue at a supermarket . . . . I'm not a bad parent, it is part and parcel of their whole condition. This gave me some reassurance, to be honest. I don't think you can predict how you will feel when you hear that difficult news.* **"**

Rachel recalls:

" *I don't know how I felt, to be honest. There was the relief that finally I had a name for the way Charlie behaves. There was the immense sadness that I had a name for it, there was anger, guilt, blame and lots more confused emotions. I suppose I looked at it as a mixed blessing really. I didn't want a diagnosis as you want your child to be perfect in every single way, yet I needed the diagnosis for my own sanity. So that I could face the world and show as well that it wasn't about me being a bad parent. I do know that communicating these feelings was very, very important for me. I needed someone who would listen to me and I just needed to sit and talk about how I was* *feeling without being judged. I was very lucky in that I have a friend who has gone through a similar experience. Other friends tried to give solutions, told me I would get over it and those comments aren't useful. I needed someone who would just sit and listen to me offload and give me a hug.* "

Ignoring what is happening to you emotionally can make these emotions more challenging in the long run. You need to communicate how you are feeling in order to move on. In Chapter 7 we explored Elisabeth Kübler-Ross's model of the 'Five Stages of Grief'. This can help you to realize that the reaction that you are feeling is a natural one.

It is important that you have people to talk to about how you feel in order to help you to cope with diagnosis and move on. You may find it easier to speak to a befriender or a parent that you meet at a support group, while others may find it easier to talk to a member of their family. Make it clear to the people that you speak to that you are not asking them for solutions or advice, you simply want them to listen to you and hear what you are saying about the way that you feel. People often want to help but are unclear as to how they can do so. Sharing your feelings with them can help you to feel less isolated. However, if your feelings become too much to cope with you must seek help from your GP.

Chloe says:

" *Talking to other parents who have been through similar things has certainly helped me. You feel so lonely at times and you think that you are the only person going through this situation. For example, the other day I went to a support group meeting and I really didn't want to go. But when I got there I found myself feeling so much better. A mum was talking about how she avoids social activities with her child and I could relate to that. A dad shared how they had been so pleased that their son had been invited to a birthday party yet when they arrived he couldn't cope with it and bit another child. I could so relate to that too! It really does help to listen to other parents and to speak to them about how your life is. When I left the support group that day I definitely felt a lot better and like I could cope more effectively once more.* **"**

Some parents draw comfort from their faith while others may question their faith in the wake of the diagnosis. Speaking to a figure within your religious community may be helpful in these situations.

Unless somebody has experienced diagnosis, they are unlikely to truly understand how you are feeling. Nobody should put pressure on you to 'get over it' or to 'move on' and neither should you put pressure on yourself. You should experience the feelings that you have without fear of judgment.

You may not feel ready to speak to others about how you are feeling; if that is the case you could consider sharing your feelings in a very different way. Some parents write a journal as a way of releasing their feelings. Perhaps you could write your thoughts down in a letter or maybe make a scrapbook that concentrates on celebrating your child's achievements and life. Some parents described how they found this really interesting to look back on. Theresa says:

" *I kept a journal when my child was going through diagnosis for autism. At the time it helped me as I was able to share my deepest thoughts about the whole process. Now I look back and I can see how much progress Dylan has made. I love reading it and seeing how he has progressed over time and also how I have progressed as well in my ability to cope.* **"**

Professionals and communication

Many parents reported that they felt that there was no follow-up support from professionals following diagnosis. Parents who had received follow-up support felt more equipped to cope. Ask the professionals involved with your child whether there will be the opportunity to meet once assessment is completed. A meeting a few weeks following diagnosis can be helpful as it can allow you the opportunity to reflect on any questions that you may have and to discuss your feelings about the diagnosis and assessment. If the professionals are unable to offer this kind of support you could ask them if they are aware of any support groups running locally where you may gain this kind of assistance.

It is interesting to note that the way diagnosis is given may have an impact on how you cope with it. A survey by Howlin and Moore in 1997 found that parents gained more satisfaction from the diagnosis process when diagnosis was carried out with less delay. Waiting for diagnosis can be extremely difficult and many parents that we discussed diagnosis with for the research for this book shared that the time element of process could be extremely stressful. Ask for clarity about timescales whether it be for a follow-up clinic or for further assessment within school. Make sure that you are aware of how long this may take and make a note of it in your diary. If you don't hear anything then contact the professionals involved to ask for an update. The survey also found that parents were more satisfied with diagnosis when the diagnosis was a firm one and did not discuss elements such as 'traits' or 'tendencies'.

Asking for help from any professionals who are involved in your child's care can be very important in helping you to move forward following diagnosis. The help that you ask for may be around your child and getting started with, for example, any programmes that will assist them in their development. If you know that your child is engaged in activities that are going to be helpful then this can be useful in keeping you focused and positive too.

Ask the professionals if there is anything that they can recommend that you do with your child in order to promote their skills. Also ask for any recommendations for materials to read so that you can educate yourself more. Initially you may feel that you have too much information; many parents that we have spoken with reported feeling overwhelmed by the amount of written information they were initially given. Over time you will feel more equipped to read this information and make sense of it – the period immediately following diagnosis may not be the right time for you to attempt to read it.

Asking for help can be difficult initially, especially if you are an independent type of person. Whether it be professionals that you ask for help or family it is very likely that these people will be keen to help you; they may just not know in what form to offer their support. You will become an advocate for your child so it is important that you know as much as possible and take advantage of any services on offer in your community.

If you are finding professionals difficult to get hold of always leave a message if they have a voicemail. When you manage to get hold of them ask them if they have a work mobile number that you may use or an email address that you can contact them on. Julie says:

I admit that I chase professionals to get the information that I want. I am pushy because I'm doing it for my daughter, not for myself. If it was for myself I would just sit and wait for the phone to ring or the next appointment letter to come through the door but it is different when it is your child. I will do whatever I can to make sure that she gets the help that she deserves and if that means that I'm regarded as a nuisance for being persistent, then so be it. I don't like feeling like I have to fight for support all the time but in my experience those who shout the loudest get seen first so I shall carry on shouting!

Couples and communication

If you are in a relationship, at times you will experience very different emotions about a range of issues. Diagnosis can be experienced very differently on an emotional level; this can lead couples to misunderstand each other and can cause arguments. Acknowledge that you are both going through a difficult time and that you both share the same objective for your child, which is for them to meet their full potential. It is also important to remind yourselves that you both love your child dearly.

Rob shares his experience:

Shelly has a son from a previous relationship who had already been diagnosed as having ADHD. She'd been through the whole process before and knew what to expect. Isabelle is my first and only child. I was devastated to think that there was anything at all wrong with her. I found the whole assessment process extremely distressing while Shelly just seemed to accept what was going on. When we received the diagnosis I went to pieces. I remember sobbing and sobbing in front of the psychologist. Shelly was completely calm and in control and I remember thinking, 'What's wrong with you? Why aren't you hurting like me?' I was quite angry to be honest at Shelly, I thought she was hard and uncaring. I now realize that she had been through this before; she was better prepared than I was. She did still feel hurt and upset but she moved through the emotions much more quickly than I was able to. It was actually Shelly that explained this to me and what she said made sense. We are fine now and I understand that we both care deeply for Isabelle. I think it is enormously confusing though when you are in a relationship and you don't understand how the other person is feeling and reacting, particularly when it relates to a child that you've brought into the world together. **"**

At times you may feel angry or even experience conflicting feelings. These emotions are normal. Try not to direct your anger at each other, however. Direct your anger towards the disorder rather than your loved one. The issue of diagnosis will be painful for both of you and will evoke strong emotions. Be very aware that if you begin to argue about issues relating to diagnosis that it is the diagnosis that is actually upsetting you, not your partner.

Ruth explains how she and her husband find it difficult to communicate:

" *Our daughter has a rare disorder, to be honest I'm not sure how I made it through those early days following diagnosis. My GP did offer me counselling as an option but I turned it down as I felt I could only function if I kept a lid on my emotions. I'm now able to talk about my daughter's difficulties but my husband can't. He gets very withdrawn if I mention it and retreats into his cave or becomes very practical and tries to offer me solutions to what he perceives the problem to be. It's not at all helpful in terms of me getting any emotional support but I know that he's doing it because this is his way of coping.* **"**

It is also interesting to note how the diagnosis may mean different things to each partner. For example, one partner may have to stay at home to care for the child while the other partner may have to work increased hours to ensure that the household remains financially stable. Life plans may have to be reviewed.

Parenthood is exhausting anyway and having a child with an additional need can increase these feelings. It may be that one parent is more involved with appointments than the other due to work factors. Many parents discussed the fact that the mother was at home with the child and having contact with professionals while the father was out at work. This can lead to difficult feelings: the mother may begin to feel overwhelmed by all the appointments, as well as feeling unsupported and resentful. On the other hand, fathers reported feeling isolated and excluded, which can lead to relationship issues if these feelings aren't discussed openly and honestly.

Generally speaking, men and women communicate using different styles and this can present challenges to relationships. Women are generally seen as being good at 'rapport talk', which includes talking, nurturing, empathy and support. Men, in contrast, are generally recognized as being experts in 'report talk'. Men typically communicate to analyze and solve problems and focus on accomplishing tasks. These different communication styles can lead parents into conflict.

Simone runs a support group and she tells us about the different styles of communication she sees:

" I've always found it difficult to engage fathers in support groups. I've tried many different approaches and eventually found that a breakfast club was the most effective in our area. On the first meeting I sat back and listened to the men communicating and I was surprised at how different the conversations were compared to when the women get together. With the mums I hear a lot of emotional support; they talk a lot about their feelings about their child, their relationship and their lives. The mums tend to really listen to each other and empathize. The dads, on the other hand, were not speaking at this same emotional level. They were offering each other support but it tended to be in a more

practical kind of way. For example, one dad needed an adaptation carrying out to his property for his son's wheelchair and the other dads immediately gave advice regarding how to go about this or who might be able to help. The information that they were sharing was factual and aimed to solve a problem. "

Gender differences in communication can have an impact on a couple. You will both be responding to the same situation but it may well be in very different ways. Mothers may want to talk about their stress while fathers generally prefer to withdraw to deal with their stress, although this will obviously vary based on individual personalities. Some mothers find 'rapport talk' a challenge just as some fathers find this more natural than 'report talk'. Whatever your situation, acknowledging these differences in communication style can help us to understand that we deal with emotions in different ways and neither is right or wrong, just different.

It is important that you spend some time on your relationship as a couple. When we have children we can find that our relationship is challenged, leaving us with less time and energy for each other. Parents often find themselves very short of time, which leaves less time to focus on their relationship. Energy levels can become depleted, which can mean that couples have less enthusiasm for sex and finances can also be put under pressure.

With the additional pressure that diagnosis may have brought, couples need to work even harder to stay connected. Enjoying a date with your other half on a regular basis is a good way to keep the relationship alive. This may not even have to involve leaving the house if you are struggling to get babysitters or if money is an issue. What it should involve is spending some quality time together on an activity that you both enjoy such as watching a movie or enjoying a favourite meal.

As we have consistently heard, talking is important to keep relationships healthy. Often parents find it challenging to talk when they are following busy schedules and leading hectic lives. Make some time each day to talk as it is vitally important for a healthy relationship. Conversations about parenting are important to keep you working as a team; conflict can appear in relationships if you are dealing with things in a different way to each other. It is important that you talk about and understand how each of you would like to handle different situations and that you then negotiate this to come to a compromise. It is, however, also important that you talk about mundane things away from the topic of work or parenting, for example, discussing a TV show or a piece of music that you have heard and enjoyed. Sex is also an important part of a relationship and physical intimacy can help you to feel connected to your partner as well as being a great stress reliever. You may find that your libido is low – later in this chapter we discuss how to alleviate stress and these tips should help.

If you feel it would be helpful you may wish to explore the option of couple's counselling. This can help you to discuss your feelings in a safe and secure environment.

Relate offers relationship counselling, which can help you to make the most of your relationships. Relate counsellors provide a caring environment where you can talk through any difficulties that you may be experiencing. To find your nearest Relate counsellor log on to their website at www.relate.org.uk. They have also published a range of self-help books, which are available on their website.

Looking after yourself

In order to look after your child effectively, you first need to look after yourself. Parents are very good at neglecting their own well-being and putting others' needs in front of their own but it is now more important than ever that you take care of yourself. Stress can deplete your energy levels very quickly.

You may not feel like eating at times but it is important to eat regular, healthy meals. Exercise can also help you to feel better and planning a walk every day can help to lift your mood. Regular exercise is one of the best methods of dealing with stress available. If you are unable to have time away from your children you could consider purchasing an exercise DVD to do at home. Or if it is possible to make exercise a family activity then take the children with you on a walk or jog. Although it may be tempting to use drugs or alcohol to cope, any mood lift that is achieved is artificial and may lead you to feel much worse afterwards.

Difficult feelings that continue

It is totally natural to feel these difficult feelings following diagnosis, but as time goes on the intensity of these emotions should begin to fade. If, however, you aren't starting to feel better or you are beginning to feel worse it may be a sign that you are suffering from depression. If sadness is taking over your life you need to speak to a health professional straight away. Signs that suggest that you should be seeking help include feeling that life isn't worth living, feeling numb and disconnected from the world and an inability to perform your normal daily activities.

Meeting all needs

It can be difficult not to become all-consumed by a diagnosis. It is, however, important to recognize that the diagnosis that you have received is a part of your life but not ALL of your life. Be aware of how much time and energy you spend on the actual diagnosis itself and finding out information. If this is getting out of proportion then make an effort to spend some time doing things that you may have done prior to diagnosis.

It can also be challenging if you have typically developing children, as meeting their needs is important too. Everyone in your family is needy of support, so here are some ideas around how to handle this.

Your child

Although your child may now have a diagnosis, acknowledge that they are still the same wonderful child that they have always been. Having a diagnosis does not define your child, what it does is change the methods that are used to work with them. Focus on what they can achieve and what they can do rather than making comparisons between them and typically developing children. It is important that you love them for who they are rather than who you had planned that they would be.

Rachel says, 'When I received the diagnosis one of the professionals said to me, "This is still the same wonderful child that you gave birth to, this is the same wonderful child as you had yesterday, your child hasn't changed, the way that we will work to meet their full potential has changed." These words gave me a lot of comfort.'

Siblings

Being the brother or sister of a child with an additional need can be challenging at times. It is important that you communicate openly and honestly with your other children about the diagnosis. Remind them that every family is faced with challenges at some point and that while the diagnosis that has been received is challenging it is a difficulty that you may face together.

If the siblings are old enough then you may wish to discuss the diagnosis with them very openly. If you are comfortable talking about it then they will learn to be comfortable talking about it too. You should also be aware that the child's school may need to be informed about the diagnosis as sometimes it can impact on the functioning of another child. The school may know of families in a similar position and may be able to introduce your child to another pupil who is going through a similar situation.

Siblings may also feel sad or have a range of other feelings about the diagnosis. Acknowledge these feelings and spend time discussing these with your children rather than avoiding them. Research suggests that siblings would like to have information about their brother or sister's condition. Consider whether this is appropriate and what sort of information you could share to help them to understand what is happening. It is important that you do share information with your other children about what is happening at a level they can understand. Also allow opportunities for them to ask questions. Make sure that they know that they can ask you if there is anything that they don't understand or anything else that they wish to know. You may wish to ask professionals to include siblings in any meetings if appropriate.

One of the biggest worries that siblings tend to have is not knowing what will happen to their brother or sister should they need full support once you as parents are unable to provide this. The information in Chapter 8 should have helped you to consider the future in a way that will ensure that forward planning can take place.

Some organizations run support groups specifically for siblings or young carers. There are condition-specific organizations that run workshops specifically for siblings to attend. You can contact the appropriate organization for your child's condition and ask them if they have information about sibling support. Sibs is an organization based within the UK for brothers and sisters of people with special needs. You can find more information about their work on their website at www.sibs.org.uk. There have also been a number of books published specifically aimed at siblings of children with additional needs that may be helpful to explore issues.

Having a child with additional needs can be time consuming for you as a parent, but your other children also need your time and need to feel important too. Find an activity that you can include all of your children in; shared activities can be important for developing family bonding. The activity may be something like baking a cake or planting some new seeds in the garden. Ask your other children for ideas about activities that you can all do together. The Sibs website has a section full of simple ideas and advice on developing positive relationships within the family unit.

Grandparents

Grandparents can be an incredible source of support for some families and some grandparents have a great deal to offer. Grandparents too may be going through a difficult emotional time acknowledging the diagnosis. It is important that they seek out their own support if this is the case.

Sharing information about the diagnosis can be helpful in the sense that the more you talk about the matter the better you can eventually feel. It may be difficult initially to talk about the diagnosis but as time goes on it should become easier.

Grandparents can also provide important support in ensuring that you have quality time with all of your children if they are willing/able to offer support in terms of care. If you feel that you can ask then suggest to them that they look after one of your children for an hour on a regular basis so that you can spend that time with the other child.

If they are concerned about looking after a child with additional needs you could suggest that they do this at your home while you are still present in another room. They can also provide an important role in giving any other children that you have vital attention to make sure that their needs are also being met fully.

Grandparents Plus is a charity covering England and Wales, which champions the vital role of grandparents. The charity operates a helpline that grandparents can call for information and advice. You can find their website at www.grandparentsplus.org.uk.

Stress management

Parenting is a stressful job and there are times when you will experience stress creeping into your life. Assessment and diagnosis can be extremely stressful periods. Stress can have a negative impact on our health and can affect our relationships and daily functioning.

Stress can manifest in all kinds of ways including having difficulty relaxing and making decisions, weight loss, sleep disturbance or increased illness. It is important that you recognize how stress impacts on you so that you can be aware if your stress levels are rising. This needs to be an ongoing process.

Different people are stressed by different things. Consider what exactly it is that is making you feel stressed: Is it having to attend meetings? Is it the prospect of a new piece of equipment being introduced to your child? Is it that your child is due to move to a different school? It could even be a culmination of lots of smaller issues that are building up and causing you to feel stressed.

Simple stress-busting strategies

There are some simple strategies that you can follow in order to manage stress in your life more effectively. Making time to relax and unwind is vitally important. Children also need time to unwind and it could be that you can initiate activities that involve you relaxing together. Listening to soothing music, enjoying a hand massage or playing a favourite game are all examples of stress-relieving activities that you could explore. Singing along to a favourite CD can be a great stress reliever. Music can be very therapeutic and take your mind away from your worries. There are a great number of relaxation CDs on the market with some aimed specifically at children – visit www.relaxkids.com to view their range. Practicing relaxation activities can really help to keep your stress levels manageable.

Hobbies are important in relieving stress and there are a great variety of hobbies that you can engage in from the comfort of your own home. Gardening, reading or craft-type activities are all things that you could engage in and will provide outlets for any stress that you may be experiencing.

Take some time to clear the clutter out of your house. An untidy living environment can make you feel stressed and can make life seem more chaotic. Take time to organize each room so that you are able to create a calm, orderly environment. Ask others to help you too, particularly if you feel that you are finding it difficult to keep up with daily chores.

Breathing exercises are simple yet highly effective stress relievers. Deep breathing is highly beneficial for the body and can help to oxygenate the blood, which will make the brain more alert. Breathing exercises can also help to relax the muscles and quieten your mind. The good thing about breathing exercises is that you can do them anywhere and nobody will notice.

Claire says:

❝ *I was taught some breathing exercises when I went on a parents' course. I didn't actually think they would work but they do. Whenever I have to go into a stressful meeting about my child now I calm myself down by doing the breathing exercises. I find that they help to make me feel more in control and they also give my mind something else to focus on.* **❞**

One simple breathing method to try can be carried out in either a relaxed standing or seated position. Slowly inhale through your nose while you count to five in your head, then let the air out through your mouth as you count to eight in your head. Repeat this several times to release tension. Some people find it helpful to imagine breathing in calmness and relaxation and breathing out their worries and anxieties.

Progressive muscle relaxation is another technique that can be used to help you to eliminate tension. By tensing up each muscle group in your body and then relaxing it you can relieve tension in minutes. Begin by tensing up your facial muscles and holding this for ten seconds before relaxing. Move on then to your neck muscles and again relax them after ten seconds. Continue this sequence for all the muscle groups around your body. As you practice you will find that you can quickly release any tension that you are holding physically within your body.

Complementary therapies

You may wish to consider complementary therapy as a way of managing your stress levels. It is estimated that 80% of all health issues are stress related. Complementary therapies offer an alternative to traditional medicine and many claim that they are helpful in reducing stress levels.

Complementary therapies can include things like Indian head massage, reiki, hypnotherapy, acupuncture and aromatherapy. You may wish to contact your local college as many put on sessions at a significantly reduced rate so that their students can practice their techniques.

Jean says:

" *I use complementary therapy to help me with my stress levels. I was introduced to it through my daughter's special school. They put on a funded session for parents and carers to experience massage. I found it incredibly relaxing and I have continued to have regular sessions to help me to unwind. I'm now learning massage and reflexology myself and hope that I will be able to set up a charity to help other carers to manage their stress levels.* "

If you find that your stress levels are becoming too high you must seek medical help from your GP.

Fundraising and charity work

Some parents find it helpful to do something that feels positive following diagnosis. This may involve raising funds for your child's school or the unit where they were treated if they have required medical care. Other families have found it helpful to set up a charity so that they can support other parents going through similar issues.

It may be worth considering what positives can come from the diagnosis for both you and your child. Are there any areas that you are interested in learning more about? Or would you like to offer some time to a charity or even set up your own support group? You do not need to do these things immediately but having thoughts about how you can progress may be helpful in your journey of moving on.

Support in education

The education system can seem very confusing when you start to look at special educational needs issues. Following diagnosis you may wish to share the information with your child's school. You should ensure that whoever makes the diagnosis also shares the information in written form with the school so that your child's teacher is clear about the diagnosis that has been made and how this will impact on your child's learning.

You may wish to request a meeting with your child's teacher following diagnosis to share with them any relevant information that has come to light. Take with you any copies of reports relating to your child's assessment so that you can refer to these as necessary.

The Code of Practice

You may find it useful to get yourself a copy of the SEN Code of Practice. This is a document that gives guidance to schools and local authorities around how to assess and support children with additional needs. You can request a free copy from the Department of Education website: www.education.gov.uk.

If your child needs a lot of additional help or resources the local authority may decide to carry out a statutory assessment of their needs. You can ask for an assessment in writing. Statutory assessment can lead to a statement of educational needs being issued.

Most children with additional needs, however, do not have a statutory assessment and their needs are met within school. If your child has been identified as having an educational additional need they will be put onto the special needs register at what is known as 'School Action'. If they do not make sufficient progress they can then be moved up to 'School Action Plus', which means that the staff need outside specialists to input, such as a speech therapist or educational psychologist. For children in early years settings these stages are referred to as 'Early Years Action' or 'Early Years Action Plus'.

If you feel that your child is not getting the right amount of support to meet their needs you should initially voice your concerns to the class teacher. If you still feel that their needs are not being addressed then you should ask to meet with the SENCO. It is important that when you have these meetings you are very clear about what you want to change. It may be helpful to consider the following:

✓ What is it exactly that you are unhappy about?
✓ Is your child making any progress?
✓ What would you like to see changing?
✓ Does your child require more intervention from specialists?
✓ Would your child benefit from having more one to one support?

Ask for a follow-up meeting to take place in a few weeks' time so that you can discuss progress that has been made and continue to work in partnership with the school to resolve any issues.

Parent Partnership

Parent Partnership services offer impartial information relating to special educational needs for parents and carers. The service can help you to understand issues relating to education and they provide a confidential service. The Parent Partnership service can be useful in explaining to you how systems work and what you should do if you continue to feel unhappy with the situation at school.

The National Parent Partnership Network exists across England and Wales. To find out where your local service is situated log on to the website at www.parentpartnership.org.uk.

Individual Education Plans

Individual Education Plans or IEPs are used to plan and evaluate how children with additional needs are learning. These documents are a way of planning the next small achievable target to support your child's development. The targets should be reviewed on a regular basis and as a parent you should be aware of what targets your child is working towards. You should also be encouraged to input into the targets and to evaluate the progress. If your child has not got an IEP but you think they would benefit from one you should contact their class teacher to see if it is something that needs to be implemented to support their learning.

Becoming assertive

Many parents shared with us that they have had to develop their communication skills as a result of their child's diagnosis. Sharon says:

" *It's been a steep learning curve for me. I used to dread going to meetings with professionals. I really have had to learn how to get my point across and to be assertive without being aggressive. I'm there representing my child and in a way that makes it easier. I'll stand up for her rights whereas I wouldn't stand up for my own. She is my inspiration. She hasn't got a voice; I am her voice. My daughter is relying on me and that spurs me on.* **"**

Being assertive is very different to being aggressive. Assertiveness means that you stand up for your point of view while still respecting the thoughts and ideas of others. Some people seem to be naturally assertive while others need to work on developing this important communication skill.

Assertive communication gives you a good method of sharing your thoughts and ideas about your child. If you give this information in a manner that is either too passive or aggressive the listener may react to your delivery rather than the information.

If you are naturally a passive person and tend to agree with the majority for a quiet life you may find yourself becoming angry and resentful if decisions are made about your child that you are not happy with. Passivity around these decisions can lead to a lot of internal conflict as you may feel guilty that you didn't share your point of view.

On the other hand, being aggressive in meetings is not an effective method of communicating or getting your child's needs met. Aggression within meetings can come across as being threatening and is likely to damage the relationships that you are trying to build up with professionals. Sarah is an early years advisory teacher and tells us:

" *I do a lot of work with families and I really do try to hear things from their point of view. I've encountered aggressive parents on a number of occasions and it is actually very intimidating and frightening. I think that they believe by being aggressive it will make professionals work harder for them and do more; it actually has the reverse effect. It makes you want to avoid them in all honesty!* **"**

Having an assertive manner can help you to remain in control while avoiding saying 'yes' to things that you don't want to agree to around your child. It can also help you to develop your self-esteem and feel more confident.

We develop our communication styles over time and you may not be aware of the style that you use. Spend some time thinking about how you are likely to respond in meetings. Do you say what you really want to say or do you tend to stay silent?

Here are some tips to help you to develop a more assertive style when in meetings:

✓ Use 'I' statements so that you own the statement and avoid blaming others. For example, saying 'I disagree with you' sounds more acceptable than telling a professional 'You are wrong'

✓ If you know that the meeting that you are attending is going to be difficult then you may find it helpful to rehearse the meeting mentally the day before. Say what you want to say out loud so that you can hear yourself actually verbalizing your thoughts and ideas. Consider writing things down to use as a prompt if necessary

✓ If a suggestion is made that you are not in agreement with then you need to say so. Sometimes you may need to practice saying 'no' if it feels uncomfortable to you. If you do feel that you need to justify why you are saying no to a suggestion, keep your reasoning brief

✓ Body language can also help us to appear assertive, even if we may not be feeling assertive. Keeping an upright posture is helpful and making eye contact is a useful strategy to adopt. Avoid fidgeting or making overdramatic gestures if you wish to appear to be in control. Be aware that your body language can make you appear to be defensive if you cross your arms or turn your body away from the speaker. Body language can also make you appear aggressive, for example, if you refuse to sit down in a meeting or if you clench your fists or put your hands on your hips; aim for a neutral pose

Developing assertiveness does take time. If you aren't naturally an assertive person then you will need to practice until you feel more confident. If, despite trying, you find it difficult to develop these skills there are many assertiveness training courses available to support you in developing these skills. By becoming assertive you can express your feelings and ideas more effectively around your child's development.

Positive thinking

Positive thinking is incredibly powerful and an important tool to use when you are trying to move on from diagnosis. Positive thinking is not about looking at life through rose-tinted spectacles or being overly optimistic. Positive thinking is a mental attitude that can help daily life move along more smoothly. You may have heard people telling you to 'think positively', which can be very challenging to do in certain situations, particularly when the situation involves your child.

Positive thinking doesn't mean that you pretend that everything is wonderful in your life. What it means is that you approach a difficult situation in a more productive and positive manner. Positive thinking begins inside your own head. We all have what we will refer to as 'self-talk' running in our minds each and every day – that little voice that gives a constant stream of orders, instructions, reminders and so on. This 'self-talk' can be positive or negative in nature. If the majority of this 'self-talk' is negative then you are likely to become a pessimist and always look at life in a negative way. However positive 'self-talk' is found more often in optimists and positive people.

Research has been conducted into positive thinking and it has been found that it has many benefits. Positive thinking has been linked to lower rates of depression and better psychological well-being and it has even been found to be beneficial to the immune system. Positive thinking is contagious and those around you will pick up on your positivity.

Developing positive thinking skills is much more involved than just telling yourself to think more positively; this thinking takes time and practice to develop. Here are some tips to help you to become a more positive thinker:

✓ When talking about your child focus on what they *can* do
✓ Use positive phrases when in meetings such as 'we will achieve' or 'it is possible'
✓ Try to disregard negative thoughts and remember: it is important to be realistic in your targets for you and your child. Any target should be achievable and it is about focusing on what *can* be done
✓ Mix with people who are positive thinkers. Negative people tend to make you feel worse about situations while positive people make you feel much better
✓ Be aware of your 'self-talk' and substitute the negative thoughts for more positive ones. Don't say anything to yourself in 'self-talk' that you wouldn't say to other people; be kind to yourself!
✓ When your child is asleep take some time to think of one thing that you love about them whether it be a quality or simply their beautiful smile. Visualize this clearly in your mind. This exercise helps you to reconnect with the positive aspects of your child
✓ Use visualization to help you to rehearse meetings going well. If you are dreading meeting the SENCO, for example, run through the meeting in your mind and visualize it as being a successful meeting, achieving the outcome that you desire. Visualizing yourself doing something greatly improves the odds of you achieving your desired goal

✓ Allow yourself to laugh and explore humour as a way of dealing with difficult situations. Julie says:

" There are some days I just laugh at the situation that I'm in. For example, my child refused to get off a bus at the bus stop. Everybody was staring, it was horrible at the time. The situation seemed to go on forever. Afterwards I reflected back and had a good old laugh about it as I imagined how I must have sounded trying desperately to remove my child from the seat whilst carrying my shopping and making an attempt to keep my dignity intact. I suppose it's a bit of black humour creeping in; if others laughed you'd be horrified but it's OK for me to laugh about it, it helps to keep me sane, I think. "

Positive thinking takes time to develop and will not happen overnight. With practice your 'self-talk' can become more positive and you can become kinder to yourself. Practicing positive thinking will help you to have an improved outlook on life following diagnosis. So how can you view a diagnosis positively? Here are a few ideas to consider:

✓ It is an opportunity to learn about a new condition
✓ You will meet some fantastic parents and children along the way who you would never have met otherwise
✓ There will be challenges that you can tackle from different angles than you may have previously considered
✓ You will develop a new appreciation for your child's abilities and successes
✓ You will acknowledge difficulties that others face in their lives with increased compassion

It would be very wrong to suggest that positive thinking is easy, particularly at difficult times. However, thinking more positively will have an impact on the way that you feel about the situation you are in and with practice can be an extremely useful tool for you to use.

Enjoying your child

It is important that you take time out to actually enjoy being a parent and enjoy spending time with your child. Consider what your child enjoys doing and perhaps build up an activity that you can share around this interest. The activity may only last a couple of minutes initially but that is fine as long as you all get some pleasure from it. Many children, for example, enjoy going swimming and specialist hydrotherapy pools are often available for disabled children to access with their families. Or it may be that your child enjoys the outdoors and an open space such as a park makes the ideal place for them to run off their energy.

Sometimes getting everything achieved in terms of looking after children and a home can seem overwhelming. You may need to give yourself permission to do less for a short period of time. Make a list of the things that you need to do and prioritize the tasks. Make a conscious effort to only do the necessaries for one day and to spend the rest of the time enjoying yourself with your child. Remember not to put pressure on yourself for everything to be perfect in your home; it is a target that few of us ever achieve.

We live in a fast-paced society where everything happens quickly yet living with a child with an additional need tends to require a slower pacing. Allow your child to set the pace. Does it matter if you are still not dressed by lunchtime on a weekend? We are constantly bombarded with texts, emails and phone calls, all of which can distract us from the here and now. Switch off your phone and computer sometimes so that there are no outside distractions or pressures on you or your time.

With so many things to do it is very easy to become distracted. Make a real conscious effort to spend quality time enjoying your child. Observe their face, any little movements they make and become engrossed in the moment rather than worrying about what you are going to cook for tea later on. Play is a wonderful way to connect with children and children with the most profound difficulties still enjoy play. Take some time alongside your child to become involved in play. It might mean dressing up, painting, hide and seek type games, whatever your child finds enjoyable. Allow yourself to really enjoy the moment and laugh alongside your child. If it is possible then take the play outdoors and enjoy the fresh air.

Slowing down and spending quality time with your child can help you to feel more connected and also calmer. When we rush around trying to be super-parents we often feel frustrated and irritable. Taking time out to enjoy our children leads to more positive feelings and a happier more fulfilling relationship between parent and child.

In summary

Enjoying your child seems to be a good place to end a chapter that has focused on moving on from diagnosis. Enjoying your child is perhaps the ultimate reward for parents. The skills that we have discussed in this chapter, including positive thinking, communication skills, developing assertiveness and dealing with stress, will all help you to be better equipped to enjoy your child more easily.

It is important to acknowledge the difficulties that assessment and diagnosis bring. It can be the most devastating time of a family's life to learn that their their child has an additional need and this should always be fully acknowledged. It also needs to be acknowledged, however, that positives may come from the situation and these need to be embraced and celebrated each and every step of the journey.

Chapter 10
The Positives about Assessment and Diagnosis

When you first begin on the journey through assessment it can seem a daunting process. It is very easy to become disheartened and to feel isolated during this time. This book aims to reduce the feelings of isolation that you may face as a parent or carer and to empower you to become a true partner with the professionals in the assessment process. We hope that this book has helped to demystify the process of assessment and offered you an insight into the journey that other parents have taken.

While it is true to say that assessment and diagnosis can be extremely stressful periods, they can also bring about positive changes in families' lives. Other parents will share their stories about how parenting a child with an additional need has enhanced their lives and led them to meet like-minded people, developing support groups and even developing careers that they would not have previously considered. We will also hear from professionals about the positives that assessment may bring and from the children themselves.

The professional's view

Vicky Robinson is an occupational therapist who believes that assessment can and should be a positive experience for both parent and child.

" *Assessment can help to gain a better understanding of a child's strengths and areas for development. Once the child's strengths are identified they can then be built upon to enable the child to meet their full potential. For example, if a child is a visual learner I am able to advise the teacher of this who can then provide pictures or handouts to complement any verbal*

instructions given in class. Assessment can also help to iden-
tify areas for development, which can then be targeted through
therapy. Again the child's strengths can be used to complement
the areas for development so, for example, if a child is strug-
gling with movement, I may use their imagination skills to input
into designing an obstacle course, which means that they are
in effect working on motor planning, and from there build in the
movement skills that I want to develop. "

Vicky also believes that assessment can give both parents and practitioners a better understanding of a child's functioning:

" *Assessment can help us to understand a child more completely.*
Why do they exhibit some of the behaviours observed? Why do
they perform tasks in a certain way? Through assessment these
questions can begin to be addressed and we can learn how to
respond to the child appropriately. For example, a child may be
getting into trouble at home or school for seemingly being
heavy handed or pulling children's hair, wandering off or
displaying poor attention skills. These behaviours can lead to
a child being labelled as 'naughty'. Through assessment an
occupational therapist can assess whether these behaviours
are as a result of sensory processing difficulties and, if so,
educate parents and practitioners about sensory processing
difficulties. Intervention can then be put into place, which will
allow the child to become calmer and happier at both home
and school. Assessment can avoid inappropriate labelling of
behaviours and highlight what the actual difficulties are and
how to support the child to meet their full potential. "

Assessment and its findings are not only helpful for school staff but
also for out of school activities. Vicky explains:

" *Assessment findings can help to equip a child for life. For*
example, if your child is having swimming lessons and has a
diagnosis of dyspraxia, it is important that the swimming
teacher is made aware of this. The swimming instructor will

then be able to research the condition if they do not already have an awareness of it and then use appropriate teaching methods so that the child can meet their full potential. Subtle changes in teaching style can make a huge difference to a child's functioning. **"**

Dr Kairen Cullen is an educational psychologist and tells us:

" *I use the term 'findings' rather than diagnosis as I am an educational not a medical doctor. I find that working closely with parents through the assessment process is important as I am constantly reviewing the information alongside them and this way they don't get any nasty surprises. What is important about the findings is what happens next. Categorization can be helpful to access support that their child needs. Most people are aware of the dangers of SEN labels. A label should only be given if needed. Following diagnosis parents should focus on their child as a unique individual.* **"**

Dr Cullen goes on to explain why assessment outcomes can be positive: 'Findings can help to ensure that provision is put in place for children to meet their needs. They can help to inform action planning and can clarify matters and inform follow-up. Findings can also give people a common language.'

Dr Louise Langman, also a clinical psychologist, tells us, 'Diagnosis is often beneficial because it can lead to an increase in the support available for your child. There may be options for access to services that can support with therapeutic intervention, better educational support, benefits and housing options, medication options and so on. Parents eventually feel that diagnosis can provide them with greater understanding of their child's behaviour.

Oliver's Story

Oliver is a 6-year-old child who was referred for assessment following a number of concerns that were raised at home and at school. Oliver's mum, Jo, explains:

❝ *Oliver was very disruptive in class and would wander around the room. He just didn't seem able to sit still, he would talk excessively, distracting the other children, and if he did sit down he would swing on his chair or lay across his desk. He always seemed to be 'on the go' and his concentration levels were very poor. Oliver is a bright little boy and answered questions in class showing that he understood what was taught but when it came to written work he showed little interest and rarely completed the tasks given. Oliver was most certainly not reaching his full potential and we as parents were very concerned about him as were the school; he was clearly falling behind with his learning. An assessment was suggested via the occupational therapy team and we welcomed it.* ❞

Oliver received an assessment and sensory processing difficulties were identified. Jo continues:

❝ *The occupational therapist was able to give information to both ourselves and the school about sensory processing difficulties, which meant that we immediately had a better understanding of Oliver's needs and problems. Strategies were also introduced to help him in the classroom so he was given a move 'n' sit cushion to use to promote active sitting. Regular breaks were also introduced throughout the day so, for example, he was given errands to run for the teacher and purposeful reasons to move such as cleaning the whiteboard and handing out books. Oliver was taught a communication system whereby he used a red flag to indicate when he felt that he needed a movement break. The outcome of this intervention has been incredibly positive. Oliver is now able to sit for longer periods and he can complete his work in a designated time. He is also keeping up with his friends and demonstrating through his written work his academic knowledge. Oliver's friendships have improved and he is a calmer, more organized and happier child. The teacher feels empowered now that she is meeting his needs and the whole class is benefiting because Oliver is on task and not disrupting their learning. Assessment can seem daunting but in our case the outcome has meant that Oliver can now meet his full potential and is a happy little boy, which is what really matters to us as parents.* "

A Child's Perspective

David is fourteen years old and has a diagnosis of Asperger's syndrome. The diagnosis was made two years ago now. David tells us:

" *It is good to know that there is a name for what I have. I do read about Asperger's syndrome because it helps me to know that other kids have the same sort of difficulties that I have. It also helps me to feel more 'normal' knowing that there is a reason for the way I do things and the way that I think.* "

Jake is eleven years old and has recently undergone a private occupational therapy assessment where he has been identified as having a postural instability that impacts on his written work.

" *I'm really pleased that there is a reason that my writing is so messy! My teachers have kept telling me to be more careful or changing the pens I use to try to get me to work more neatly. They just wouldn't believe me when I said that I couldn't help it. Now I have had the assessment I use a pen that helps me to write more neatly and also I have a slanted table to write on, which helps too but most importantly the teachers have stopped getting on at me about my writing, which means I'm much happier at school.* "

Developing qualities

Parenting a child with an additional need requires all kinds of skills; patience, determination, information gathering and organizational skills to name but a few. Many parents that we spoke to during our research for this book shared with us that one of the positives about assessment and diagnosis was the development of their own personal skills.

Sharon has a son who was diagnosed with autism and tells us:

" *I think I'm more consistently patient now. I'm definitely more confident. I've had to come out of my comfort zone and push for what my son is entitled to at times. I've always been a patient and non-judgmental person, but I don't think that you can truly understand what having a disabled child means until you have one of your own. I have made a real effort to educate myself about autism and am currently working in the field. I feel I have a lot to offer other parents who are going through the same as we did.* "

Danielle agrees that she has also developed as a person following her child's assessment and diagnosis with Asperger's syndrome/high-functioning autism. She says:

" *I most definitely feel that I have developed as a result of the assessment process. I am 100% more assertive. I have had to learn how to handle myself in meetings with professionals. At my son's last statement review there was myself and nine professionals in the room. I am now able to clearly share my concerns and challenge decisions that I feel are wrong. I have also become very aware that in the world of special educational needs being quiet and waiting for help to come to you doesn't work. My confidence in my parenting ability has grown. At times I have fought tooth and nail for my child; my proudest achievement to date is that I have actually got a diagnosis and statement for my son against the advice of the school who at that time had labelled him as simply being badly behaved.* "

James has a son with complex needs and shares:

" *I was not really aware of additional needs prior to my son being born. I used to see children using wheelchairs and so on but I never really stopped to think about what their lives must be like or how their parents coped. Now that I have my own child with difficulties I am much more aware. I think that I appreciate the simpler things more in life. When I'm at work and I listen to my friends talking about going out and socializing it seems like a different world that they are living in. When I finish work I go straight home and take over from my wife to give her a break. I never thought that this was how life would turn out but there are some huge positives about it. I've met some great dads who are in a similar situation to me through the local support group. I'm not sure that I'd have developed such close friendships with other dads if my son didn't have these needs. We understand how hard life can be and we offer each other support in whatever way we can. Usually it is in a practical way rather than emotionally although on the odd occasion one of us will need to offload and talk about how things are at home and the release that having that support offers is fantastic. I suppose as well I am more in touch with my emotions too. Prior to having my son I would have kept things bottled up and would have found it hard to talk about how I am feeling. I'm certainly a much nicer person now than I was. I have time for people and realize how precious life is. So there have been many positives along the process for me personally and I'm sure that will continue. It is also so important to focus on the positives, no matter how small they may seem; this is what has got me through the difficult times. It would be easy to get down and depressed about our situation but keeping in mind all the positives about life helps to keep us on track and to enjoy our time as a family.* 〃

Ria tells us:

❝ *Life is so much slower paced now that I have a child with an additional need. I used to rush, rush, rush all the time; having a job and a family there was no time to waste. Chelsea has changed all that though, she simply can't rush and I have had to learn to slow down and be patient. This has been a huge positive for me as I was living life at such speed that I was missing out on the simple pleasures. It takes Chelsea a long time to get from the house to the car for, example, and now I use this time to listen to the birds singing or to notice the flowers that are starting to bloom, all things that I simply didn't have time to observe before. Sometimes I have to remind myself to be positive. It would be so easy to think negatively and moan about how long it takes Chelsea to do things, but what would that achieve? It would make the whole situation seem worse. Thinking positively is a skill that I have developed over time and I am now a much more positive person than I ever was before Chelsea came into my life.* 〃

Understanding needs

Assessment can also bring about a greater understanding around why a child is functioning in a certain way and this in itself can bring reassurance, not only to the child but also to the parent.

Understanding her son's needs was key to Claire gaining support for her son:

❝ *For me, assessment has been positive as I have been able to get the specific help and support that my son needs. For him the biggest positive was in understanding why he found certain things difficult and that wasn't because there was something 'wrong' with him. The school are able to a degree to work around his specific needs now, which means that his anxiety levels are lower. Assessment and diagnosis has also allowed me to access support for his brother who is a keen member of our local Young Carer's group, meaning that he can now get respite and there is somewhere he can talk if he needs to. I also get support from a local support group who have been fantastic. They have picked me up when I was on the floor and supported me during the more difficult times. They really are angels in human form!* **"**

Suzanne's son has a visual impairment:

" *When Lewis was in Foundation 2 he used to get sent home flashcards to learn and he knew them without a problem. Every time school tested him, however, he appeared not to know them at all. I was very confused as to what was going on and in all honesty thought that he might have been fooling around with the teachers. His reading started to fall behind and he was getting increasingly frustrated. At a routine eye test it emerged that he had visual problems. What was happening was that the school were giving him blue flashcards during the test whereas he had white flashcards at home. Lewis could not see the text against the blue background. As soon as the teachers used white cards with him he knew them and his self-esteem started to be built back up bit by bit. I feel terrible now in the fact that I doubted him and am so thankful that I got his eyes assessed. Now if he doesn't grasp something that is visual I will always check that he can actually see it first. I'm getting much better at spotting what he won't be able to see and so are the staff at his school.* **"**

In Lewis's case assessment has led to him having increased feelings of self-esteem now that he can complete the task asked of him. It was also beneficial in avoiding him being labelled inappropriately as a child who was being deliberately difficult or challenging.

In contrast to Lewis, whose difficulties were assessed relatively early, we now turn to Tom who did not receive assessment as a child but wishes that he had. Tom has struggled all his life with feelings of anxiety and issues around socialization:

" *I was just described at school as an 'oddball', whatever that means. I was the boy who didn't fit in. I never had any friends but actually that was fine as I preferred solitary activities. I'm forty-three now and the anxiety has continued throughout my life. I have never had a relationship and avoid social situations. I do, however, have a job that I can find very stressful at times. I seek out activities such as stamp collecting or computing so that I don't have to interact with others. When I got to forty I decided that it was time to do something about this anxiety and I visited my GP. I was sent for counselling which in itself I found very difficult to attend due to my worries. I did, however, go and met a wonderful counsellor who really took time to listen to how I felt. It was actually the first time in my life I had ever shared this information and it really helped just to talk about it. One of the things we talked about at length was whether having a label for my difficulties would be useful and I considered that it would. After a while she suggested that I go back to my GP and request an assessment for social communication difficulties. I did this and earlier this year was diagnosed with Asperger's syndrome. This has really helped me to move forwards with my life. I now understand that I'm not an 'oddball' as I was described or weird, or a freak or any of the other labels I've been given throughout my life. I now understand why I feel the way that I feel and why I behave how I behave. Assessment has been incredibly helpful for me and I now have some useful strategies in place to reduce my anxiety levels. I just wish that I'd been assessed as a child.* **"**

Susan feels that assessment around transition to adult services has brought positives for her and her daughter:

" *The assessment process has identified and clarified my daughter's current additional needs. This identification of needs has made it easier for the day facility staff to get to know* *her better. It has also produced one document, which has been distributed to all stakeholders so that there is continuity for her. The document has also been useful in that it has given me a tool to prove what my daughter's additional needs and disabilities are to agencies like the Department of Work and Pensions in order to support her benefit applications.* **⁋⁋**

The social versus medical model

There are a number of different 'models' of disability but the two most commonly referred to are the 'social model of disability' and the 'medical model of disability'. Here we will examine what both of these models are and how an assessment can help in achieving the more preferred way of working.

The medical model of disability

The medical model views the disability as being the 'problem'. The disability is seen as being the concern of the individual rather than of society. The medical model focuses on the disability and attempting to 'fix' it rather than making attempts at inclusion. For example, if a building is inaccessible to a wheelchair user the medical model would consider that this is the fault of the wheelchair rather than the building design.

The social model of disability

The social model of disability is a much more inclusive model and takes the view that society has the responsibility of removing barriers to inclusion. This is an expansive model that seeks out solutions to barriers of inclusion with the onus being on the organization and society to change. So, for example, in the case of the wheelchair user being unable to access a building, the social model would look for solutions to that problem in terms of building a ramp or providing alternative access.

Organizations are now more willing to make adjustments for those with additional needs. However, those who have disabilities that are not so apparently obvious such as social communication disorders may find that the assessment process is helpful in making these needs apparent. The social model emphasizes that the individual is the expert on their requirements and that this must be respected.

Considering the positives

Sometimes it is necessary to take some time to reflect on the positives that assessment has brought in order to reassure yourself that the path you have chosen around assessment was the correct one for you and your child. Take a few minutes to consider how assessment has benefited:

✓ You – considering how you may have developed any new skills, friends or support mechanisms along the way. Also whether you have developed new knowledge about special needs or your child's condition

✓ Your relationship – if you are in a relationship, consider how assessment may have helped to strengthen this. Many couples report that they realize during these difficult periods how important their relationship is or how supportive their partner is

✓ Your child – have they received any specialist support or equipment to help them to meet their full potential? Or do they have increased self-esteem now that they know that there is a reason for the problems that they have been experiencing?

✓ Siblings – if you have other children, how have they benefited from the assessment process? Siblings can often become a forgotten group who can be greatly affected by a child's additional needs. Sharing information with siblings about assessment findings is extremely important and can help them to understand their brother or sister's functioning. There are also some support groups set up for siblings of children with additional needs, so it is worth exploring whether there is one in your area and whether your child may like to attend. Contact www.sibs.org.uk for more information

✓ Wider family/friends – sometimes having a diagnosis can be helpful to share with others outside of your immediate family as this can give them some information as to why your child functions in this way and perhaps some ideas on how they should deal with certain behaviours or issues

✓ Teaching staff – consider whether your child's school have made changes to ensure that your child meets their full potential based on the assessment findings. If so how have these changes helped your child? How might they help future students in similar situations?

Positives around people

Many of the parents that we have spoken to whilst conducting our research for this book have spoken fondly of the people that they have met during their journey through assessment. These may have been professionals who have gone that extra mile to offer support, strangers who have become friends or other parents who really understand what life can be like.

One thing that we know about assessment is that it generally leads you to meet various professionals and other parents along the way.

June's son was assessed at a very early age and she says, 'There are always positives to be found and assessment in particular has given us access to services that we need. We have also met some amazing people along the way.'

Rachel says:

❝ *My daughter draws people to us. For example, we met another couple who had a child with learning difficulties as we were walking along the sea front. The children immediately engaged with each other and we ended up chatting like you do. We shared so many common issues that we swapped numbers and five years on we are now very good friends.* ❞

Enjoying your child

Deborah's daughter has complex needs and here she tells us about how she enjoys her child:

❝ *I feel that I was born to be Annie's mother and I really appreciate the things that many parents take for granted. I think this means that I'm able to enjoy her development more. Instead of taking the developmental milestones for granted I just enjoy*

" *the wonder of her development as it emerges. A smile from her makes my day and all other problems just seem to fade away. She is an utter joy and she has taught me so much about life and not to take anything for granted. It's a real privilege to have her in our lives.* "

Veronica says:

" *My son sees the world so simply yet so brilliantly at times. He notices things that I might not see because I'm so busy, yet he points them out to me. He sees the beauty in the world, the colours . . . all the things I miss! He is so full of enthusiasm and so keen to experience the world. Above all, he is happy and what more could a parent wish for than that?* "

Diane speaks with huge fondness about her son:

" *He is beautiful, I wouldn't change him for the world. He is such a lovely boy and I am so very proud of him. He melts everybody's heart when we are out and about, in fact, he draws people to us and I've met an awful lot of lovely people through him that otherwise I would have just passed by in the street.* "

The future

Many parents shared with us how their experience of assessment and diagnosis had led them on to develop further skills and sometimes even seek out new work opportunities.

Rachel says, 'I have learned a lot through the whole process and developed my personal qualities. I now work in a school with children with special educational needs and I also volunteer with the Samaritans.'

Another mum shared her experience of becoming a volunteer as a direct result of her son's additional needs. Nicholas is nine years old and has a verbal diagnosis of Asperger's syndrome. The family are currently waiting for a formal diagnosis. Anne tells us:

“ *Nicholas has experienced social difficulties, which became particularly noticeable at school and his teacher suggested joining the Beavers to help his skills to develop. He had difficulties taking turns and found not being in control of games a challenge. When he was six years old I decided to take him and at first I didn't feel comfortable leaving him there because he needed prompting to do simple things like join in with the games or to stand still. I decided to join the parent rota and started helping out every week. This continued when he moved up into Cubs at the age of eight and I really enjoyed helping out. I was actually a keen Brownie and Girl Guide as a child! Now that he is older he is far more used to the routines and rules at Cubs and it has definitely helped him to develop and form new friendships with fellow Cubs at school. When my younger son was ready to start Beavers the waiting list was huge and I couldn't find a group for him to join so I decided to start my own. I doubt that I would have been so involved had it not been for Nicholas needing the additional support. Without him I'm sure that I would have just dropped and run like every other parent does each week. By volunteering, however, I have made a lot of friends in the Scouting world, which then prompted me to become a leader. I imagine that I will continue to volunteer well beyond my son's time in scouting and this is all thanks to Nicholas!* **”**

Emma Dawson's son has complex needs and also experienced sleep issues. Many children with additional needs also have sleep problems. Her experience as a sleep-deprived parent has led her to set up a social enterprise covering the north-east and North Yorkshire called 'SleepSense'. The organization provides sleep support to parents and training around sleep issues when a child has an additional need. Emma shares with us her inspiring story:

“ *I believe that sleep is the foundation for everything – physical, mental and emotional well-being. I know that when I was sleep-deprived I was unable to tackle the other important things in life. Sleep really is at the core of your well-being. I* *was offered some sleep counselling at a time when I really was in need and the sleep programme that the practitioners provided me with enabled me to tackle the problem with my son's sleep and gave me my strength back to take on other challenges in my life. I know how hard it is for parents and their children to function when they aren't getting the sleep they need. Unfortunately there is still very little support for parents who have sleep issues so when I realized how effective a behavioural and cognitive approach to sleep issues could be I wanted to learn more. I decided to train to become a sleep practitioner so that I could help other parents who may be in the same position that I once was. Once your child begins to sleep and you get the sleep that you need you can function so much more effectively. My son needed me to be able to function to the best of my ability in order to meet his needs fully; he was depending on me. I know how overwhelming everything feels when you are sleep-deprived and so I'm really passionate about the work that I do through SleepSense as I know that I am making a real difference to the lives of parents and children throughout the region. It's also really helpful that I've had the experience with my son as I have real empathy for those parents that I support. I can say to them that I really do know what it's like and I'm living proof that the techniques used are highly effective.* **"**

For more details about the organization visit the website at www.sleep-sense.co.uk.

Robert is the brother of Charles who has Down's syndrome. Robert explains how his brother has inspired him in his work.

" *Charles is ten years younger than me and I remember him being born very clearly. Charles is a real inspiration to me and always has been; he has found it more challenging to meet developmental milestones but he showed such determination as a youngster that I held a great admiration for him. I felt a great sense of pride in sharing his achievements; I watched him perform in a show at the local theatre and it was wonderful to see him up on that stage alongside his friends. I decided to* *train as a teacher and felt drawn to working with children with special needs. I'm sure that this is all down to Charles and the joy he's given me throughout our lives. As Charles was growing up I met some of the professionals involved with him and was touched by their dedication. I now work as a special school teacher and think that living in a family where there has been a child with special needs has really helped me to understand what home life can be like at times.* 🙶

Lynne talks about how her son has inspired her:

🙶 *How has my son inspired me? That's a huge one. I think I've been fascinated and intrigued with autism since he was diagnosed. There's so much that we still don't know so I made it a priority to educate myself so that I could better understand and help him. Prior to having him I worked as a director level PA, and I have an Honours degree in Business Studies.*

One thing that struck me over the years though was the lack of support for parents after they are given a diagnosis. I knew I wanted to be involved in autism in some way, but knew I couldn't deal with kids on the spectrum all day then have energy to deal with my son at home afterwards. Supporting parents seemed to be a good alternative and I was debating doing a counselling course when the job that I now have was advertised.

My job title is 'Project Manager' and I work for a charity called ADHD & Autism Support Harrow who support parents/carers of people with a diagnosis of ADHD and/or autism. We hold coffee morning support groups, parenting courses etc. My job involves dealing directly with the parents and I facilitate the SCATT (Supporting Carers of Autism Through Training) course, which is a course that educates parents on the basics of autism. I'm still utilizing my previous skill set too by being involved in funding bids and administrative tasks.

I believe that you can better support parents when you can truly understand what they are going through. I think parenting my son has made me a more patient and less judgmental person. It's also taught me to appreciate the small things. 🙷

The contact details for the charity can be found at www.adhdandautismharrow.co.uk.

In summary

Although assessment and diagnosis can be a very challenging time for all concerned there are often positives that can come out of it. These positives can be in the short term with pieces of equipment being offered to help your child to meet their full potential, for example, or perhaps in the longer term, by inspiring you to follow a different career path or set up a support group.

Embracing the positives is challenging at times, yet it is essential in order to ensure that the journey through assessment is as productive as possible for you and your child. Parenting can be an extremely difficult job, and it is important to remember to be kind to yourself and to celebrate the achievements that you and your child have made. Finally, have faith in yourself and remember that *you* are the expert on *your* child.

Index